"Honest and wise like Zen itself—Ronna Kabatznick's words give straightforward, clear lessons for all who struggle with food. The awareness and kindness of these teachings offer every eater sound advice and the greatest miracle of all—a change of heart." —JACK KORNFIELD, author of *A PATH WITH A HEART*

"Ronna Kabatznick's reverence for food is one of the most fascinating aspects of *The Zen of Eating*. She reminds us to pause before eating to marvel at the abundance and variety of food before us, to honor the many hard-working people who contributed to putting each ingredient on the table, to give a thought for people everywhere that they may have enough food for the day, and to eat and enjoy our food. Dr. Kabatznick's experiences feeding hungry people in California soup kitchens enriches the book in many ways." —FRANCES M. BERG, M.S., author of *AFRAID TO EAT: CHILDREN AND TEENS IN WEIGHT CRISIS*, editor and publisher of *HEALTHY WEIGHT JOURNAL*, licensed nutritionist, and Family Wellness specialist

"Ronna Kabatznick, a longtime mindfulness practitioner, uses the Buddha's basic teaching of awareness and liberation from suffering to transform the task of weight-management from struggle to spiritual journey." —SYLVIA BOORSTEIN, author of *THAT'S FUNNY, YOU DON'T LOOK BUDDHIST*

THE ZEN
OF EATING

ANCIENT ANSWERS

TO MODERN WEIGHT PROBLEMS

RONNA KABATZNICK, PH.D.

A PERIGEE BOOK

A Perigee Book
Published by The Berkley Publishing Group
A division of Penguin Putnam Inc.
375 Hudson Street
New York, NY 10014

First edition: March 1998

Published simultaneously in Canada.

The Penguin Putnam Inc. World Wide Web site address is
http://www.penguinputnam.com

Library of Congress Cataloging-in-Publication Data
Kabatznick, Ronna.
The zen of eating : ancient answers to modern weight problems /
Ronna Kabatznick.—1st ed.
p.   cm.
"A Perigee Book."
Includes bibliographical references and index.
ISBN 0-399-52382-0
1. Weight loss—Religious aspects—Zen Buddhism.   I. Title.
RM222.2.K141998
613.2'5—dc21   97-23778
                                                        CIP

Printed in the United States of America

10

This book is dedicated to

Jeffrey Kabatznick, my brother
Norman Kabatznick, my father

May their memories be for a blessing

and to

hungry people everywhere

May all beings have enough to eat

One who knows "enough is enough" always has enough.
—*Tao Te Ching*

CONTENTS

❂

ACKNOWLEDGMENTS

I have been very blessed with the support I've been given to write this book. I am extremely grateful to the many people who have generously provided it.

My literary agent, Sharon Friedman, is simply a gem. Her faith in this project and her intelligent advice throughout it have been great gifts. Amy Hertz generously helped organize my thinking within the framework of the Four Noble Truths. Suzanne Bober, my editor, provided the perfect combination of freedom and encouragement. John Duff, Dolores McMullan, and Erin Stryker helped handle the gritty details involved in creating a book.

Elizabeth Adler's many talents and wisdom graced nearly every word on every page. She generously offered valuable editorial suggestions throughout the manuscript. Her knowledge and commitment to Buddhism coupled with her unique ability to help clarify complex ideas have been enormously helpful and greatly appreciated.

Once the manuscript was in place, Barbara Gates applied her industrial-strength intelligence, inquiring mind, and beautiful heart to help me deepen the key messages in this book. As a developmental editor, she examined the structure of the book and encouraged me to express my most authentic voice.

I am particularly indebted to the precious gift of knowledge that all of my teachers have given me. Although the late Stanley Milgram wasn't a Buddhist, he had the heart of a Buddha. His respect and interest in the varieties of ordinary human experience have shaped the way I think and live my life. Stanley Keleman's insights and compassion will always be a guiding light. My primary meditation teachers and dear friends, Jack Kornfield and Gil Fronsdal, are both treasures. Their useful feedback on the historical and technical information in this book is especially appreciated.

Brian Kabatznick, Marina Bear, Zeena Janowsky, Lisa and Ed Schmidt, Joyce Block, Catherine Censor Shemo, Alison Jordan, Nancy Rothschild, Denise Silver, Judith Stronach, Marilyn Rinzler, Marilyn Lundberg, Hilda Kessler, Jane Baraz, Dan Ellsberg, Norma Kaufman, Naomi Schwartz, Catherine and Bart Gershbein, the Sax-Bolder family, the women in my meditation group, and the members of my Shabbat group are friends extraordinaire.

I owe a deep debt of gratitude to all the people I have worked with over the years who have shared their food stories and struggles with me. It has been an honor and a great gift to be part of your lives. May you be happy and peaceful.

Peter Dale Scott, my husband and best friend, is a prince. To write a first book with an established author and poet cheering me on has been the greatest blessing of all. I thank him for being who he is—a fountain of love, nourishment, and inspiration. My cup runneth over.

INTRODUCTION

◎

*And I discovered that profound truth, so difficult to perceive,
difficult to understand, tranquilizing and sublime, which is not to
be gained by mere reasoning, and is visible only to the wise.*
—THE BUDDHA

The key to healthy eating is learning how to change your state of mind. What you eat or don't eat is not nearly as important. That's *The Zen of Eating* in a nutshell.

This book is not the latest "get thin quick" plan. There are no promises or guarantees. In fact, nothing in this book is new. The wisdom found here is ancient. *The Zen of Eating* is an invitation to transform the emotional hungers that create eating problems into spiritual nourishment that creates inner peace. This kind of nourishment comes from connecting to your deepest longings and most passionate desires with wisdom and compassion. Just as millions of people have done for more than 2,500 years, you, too, can learn how to be filled with the greatest joy and peace that come from a change of heart.

The Zen of Eating is based on the teachings of the Buddha, also called *The Great Physician and Healer*. Although the Buddha isn't known as an authority on eating problems, his expertise on hungers of the heart and disorders of desire is unsurpassed. These emotional hungers are the cause of many severe problems, including alcohol and drug addictions. Like these other addictions, eating problems express both the depth and range of suffering that occurs when emotional needs are ignored and physical needs are indulged. When we focus on the fleeting pleasures that come from indulging the senses, other aspects of ourselves become deprived. The Buddha's aim was to find a way to nourish those parts of ourselves that are capable of experiencing lasting satisfaction.

The Buddha defined suffering as a ravenous appetite to find peace and security in places where it can't be found. In the context of eating, this peace and security might be sought through what you weigh, what you look like, how you cook, or what restaurants you eat in. His plan to address this ravenous appetite and to offer peace of mind and heart is known as the Four Noble Truths.

THE FOUR NOBLE TRUTHS

The essence of the Four Noble Truths and its application to your eating problems is this: Food for the body is necessary, of course, but it is eaten one day and eliminated the next, whereas food for the heart lasts forever. In fact, you can think of the Four Noble Truths as recipes for nourishing the heart, because that's exactly what they are. They address the various kinds and levels of spiritual food that are capable of providing a sense of fullness that no amount of food can ever match. The nourishing aspects of this kind of food aren't always obvious, and they contradict what many of us consider common knowledge. For instance, restraining from pleasure is more nourishing than pursuing it; generosity is more nourishing than self-indulgence; letting go of the things you love is more nourishing than grasping them.

The Four Noble Truths identify the problem, offer a diagnosis, state the outcome, and lay out the treatment plan to end suffering. Unlike traditional weight loss plans that focus on what you can take in, this plan focuses on what you can give away. It emphasizes the deep and lasting emotional satisfaction that comes from being generous, expressing gratitude, and finding special meaning and purpose in what you eat. Eating becomes a doorway to many penetrating insights that reveal the interconnectedness of all living things. Healing your own emotional hunger helps heal everyone else's as well. Just as Isaac Newton explained physical motion in three simple laws, the Buddha explains our nature in four simple principles.

Here's a brief summary of the Four Noble Truths and how they relate to eating problems:

1. *There is suffering* (the problem). The First Noble Truth recognizes that life is fundamentally unsatisfying because it is fragile. Nothing lasts. What you weigh or what you eat cannot provide lasting nourishment because they are always changing.

2. *The cause of suffering is attachment to desire* (the diagnosis). The Second Noble Truth recognizes the cause of suffering as the misguided tendency to grasp pleasure and to reject pain. But the more you grasp (or reject), the more you suffer and feel hungry. Emotional hunger grows deeper and more painful the more you struggle against it.

3. *Suffering ends by letting go of attachments to desire* (the prognosis). The Third Noble Truth recognizes that freedom from suffering is possible. It is attained by letting go of attachments to desire, which bind you to the futile habit of seeking nourishment where it cannot be found. What provides the fullness you hunger for is not grasping at what's pleasant or rejecting what isn't, but staying present with whatever is going on.

4. *The Noble Eightfold Path outlines how to let go of attachments, and so end suffering* (the treatment plan). The Fourth Noble Truth contains the recipes for emotional nourishment that offer lasting satisfaction. The skills and qualities you learn on this path are the food for the heart that the Buddha was referring to when he said that this type of food lasts forever.

The nourishment that comes from being kind to yourself and to others is the kind of food that stays with you. Unlike physical nourishment that comes and goes no matter how many times you feel full, the fullness that comes from facing difficulties head-on creates a secure foundation of confidence and self-respect that money can't buy and physical food can't give. Qualities such as personal integrity, kindness, and honesty are priceless and can only be found within your own heart. The Eightfold Path shows the various ways to access and manifest these qualities in your everyday life, no matter what you are doing or how you are feeling.

I will take you through the Four Noble Truths, step-by-step, and show you how each truth applies to your eating difficulties and how you can learn to relate to these difficulties differently. Regardless of your individual eating and weight-related struggles, the Four Noble Truths can help you understand what they are, why they exist, and how you can free yourself from them. At the end of each chapter there are questions and exercises that will further help you understand the value of the Four Noble Truths and their application to your eating problems.

MINDFULNESS DOES CURE

Mindfulness is the natural capacity for observation and reflection. It means paying attention with a spirit of kindness and acceptance to whatever is present, moment by moment. Of all the awareness practices that have been taught, mindfulness is one of the most important. It is often referred to as the medicine that cures the disease of desire. Instead of feeling depleted and deprived (as is often the case when you're trying to lose weight) mindfulness brings a feeling of nourishment and abundance. When you're not grasping, you allow the presence of awareness to breathe and fill that empty, hungry space that never feels satisfied.

Millions of Westerners over the past twenty-five years have used mindfulness to help improve their lives. Athletes, businesspeople, musicians, cancer patients, and recovering addicts are among those who have found this valuable skill enormously useful. And the numbers are growing as more and more people discover the power and potential of mindfulness. This method is the antidote to desire and the diseases that come from grasping it.

THE HUNGER FOR FULLNESS IS NOT NEW

Nobody handed the Buddha the Four Noble Truths. He discovered them for himself, just as you and I must do for ourselves. Although his life was unique in many ways, he suffered and wanted lasting happiness just like every other human being.

Born a prince, the Buddha lived a life of great luxury for his first eighteen years. He was surrounded by beauty, abundance, love, and comfort. Even without all the modern conveniences and luxuries so many of us have become accustomed to, the Buddha had it made. Every desire he had was met; every pleasure he wished for was granted.

In spite of these external comforts and delights, the young man felt empty inside and longed for a feeling of wholeness that he couldn't sustain by pleasure alone. So the Buddha left his princely life to seek a more lasting fulfillment.

Then the Buddha did what you and I have done many times. He went to the opposite extreme. Instead of indulging himself, he deprived himself. The Buddha became so thin he could touch his spine by pressing his finger on his navel. After living an austere life for six years, the Buddha abandoned it. He realized that this life of self-denial only weakened his body and mind. His hunger for inner peace was not nourished by either extreme of indulgence or deprivation. Yet his problem of how to find lasting happiness and emotional fullness remained unresolved.

THE MIDDLE WAY

Unlike you and me, the Buddha did not bounce back and forth between the extremes of indulgence (overeating) and deprivation (restricted eating). He realized that either extreme was a painful and unproductive path. Yes, he did have some glorious moments, but they didn't completely dispel his desire for lasting peace and security. You've probably had your share of blissful moments, too (great food, great sex, wonderful vacations). But when it's over, it's over, and then you find that the same old empty feeling is still there.

Instead of looking anywhere else, the Buddha decided to follow the Middle Way, to stay focused in the present moment instead of looking for extreme solutions outside himself. He turned his attention inward and mindfully examined what was going on in his own body and mind.

The Buddha sat down under a bodhi tree. He resolved not to get up until he found freedom from the hunger that seeks satisfaction where it cannot be found. During the night armies of desire, lust, pleasure, pain, aggression, fear, temptation, frustration, hatred, and doubt tried to divert him, but he was unmoved. The longer he sat, the stronger and more demanding these forces became.

Imagine sitting under a tree tantalized by your favorite sights, tastes, smells, and sounds, and then you are viciously attacked by what you most hate and find unspeakably repulsive. Imagine sitting there hour after hour, having resolved not to get up until you are absolutely certain you have discovered the key to happiness. That's exactly what the Buddha did on the evening of his enlightenment.

From the outside, the Buddha's response to these forces was unremarkable. He just sat there. But what he did on the inside was extraordinary. He focused his attention on what was going on, but he did not react to it. Sometimes the forces of desire became so strong that the Buddha had to touch the ground as his witness and support. No matter what appeared—from the most heavenly to the most demonic—he just sat there quietly and observed. He neither grasped at the delights nor rejected the repulsive. He watched them follow their natural cycle of arising and passing away without interfering with them. What he realized was as simple as it was profound. When he didn't grasp at pleasure or push away pain, he saw that his assailants were powerless. And so these forces were defeated.

By looking deeply within himself, the Buddha freed his mind from the tyranny of desire. This same freedom is available to you when you look within. What the Buddha saw and learned on that night is just as available to you and me as it was to him. He found the nourishment he was looking for, but it took both effort and honesty. There were many things he had to face and learn about before he reached enlightenment and found freedom from suffering.

He realized the lifetimes of misery that had been created because of a basic misperception: that pleasure can last and pain can be avoided. We hurt ourselves and others over and over again by grasping at experiences that change, such as our bodies and our relationships. Some suffering is inevitable because loss and change are built in to every life, but a lot of suffering is optional. It is created by our resistance to the present moment and the fact that whatever it is, it is destined to change, whether we like it or not. In fact, there's nothing to like or dislike. When you look closely at each moment, you find that opposites like pleasure and pain and even weight gain and weight loss have both advantages and drawbacks.

When you lose weight, you may feel happy for a while, but then worry sets in. You think, "What if I can't keep the weight off?" or "What if I regain it all back, or even more?" And if you gain weight, you may be upset for a while, but then a feeling of optimism may pop up. You think, "Maybe I can lose weight and feel better about myself." Weight gain and weight loss both contain elements of happiness and unhappiness, so there's no point in clinging to one and rejecting the other. They are contained within each other. When you do realize this truth based on your own experience, you can receive nourishment from any moment, regardless of its content.

The Four Noble Truths and the Eightfold Path teach you how to make peace with the challenges and changes that are always present. They explain how to let go of the infatuation with pleasure and the fear of pain so you can enjoy food, your body, and your life situation, whatever that may be now, knowing that it will eventually change. When you apply these instructions and suggestions mindfully, you learn to accept the truth of each moment graciously, without struggle. That's how you find nourishment in the places where it can be found. This is your challenge and practice, pure and simple.

INDULGENCE, RESTRICTION, AND THE MIDDLE WAY

The Buddha compared the Middle Way that you learn from applying the Four Noble Truths to a log floating down a river. On one bank is indulgence, and on the other is deprivation. As the log flows down the river, it passes both extremes. If it gets stuck on either extreme, the log sinks or rots. But when the log follows the Middle Path, it floats down the river and reaches the ocean of freedom.

Most people struggling with eating issues are stuck on the bank of either indulgence or restriction. On the bank of indulgence, fifty-eight million people in this country are defined as obese, and that number is growing. One in three Americans weighs 20 percent more than his or her ideal body weight.

On the bank of restriction, sixty million people are trying to lose weight. Although there are plenty of get-thin-quick solutions, statistics show that people are gaining more weight and losing less.

Both extremes involve a lot of suffering. Overweight people are at an increased risk for diabetes, hypertension, heart disease, stroke, gout, and some forms of cancer. Those stuck on the bank of deprivation to the point of anorexia or bulimia risk disturbing their digestive and elimination systems and even face the possibility of death by starvation. There is tremendous emotional suffering taking place at both extremes. People feel like worthless failures, unable to overcome their struggle with managing their appetites or relentless feelings of deprivation.

Unfortunately, it's not hard to figure out why finding the Middle Way of eating is so difficult for so many people. The messages we receive are as extreme as they are contradictory.

Compare, for example:

• The lucrative dieting industry and the high-fat food industry
• Frantic workdays ended with couch potato nights in front of the television
• Prepackaged diet drinks and meals like Slim Fast and Lean Cuisine next to super-size portions of fries and burgers
• Articles that say "diets don't work" with ones that promise that "this diet does."

It's up to each of us to recognize these extremes, just like the Buddha did on the night of his enlightenment. He observed and watched what appeared before him, no matter what it was. He didn't get seduced by the pleasures or betrayed by the pains because he stayed focused on the present moment without grasping or clinging. Keep in mind, the Buddha never said, "The end of suffering is easy." He did say, "The end of suffering is possible." By learning to look within and living a life of kindness and integrity, you can realize the Four Noble Truths for yourself as the Buddha did more than 2,500 years ago. These realizations and the changes that come from them are far more satisfying than anything you'll ever put in your mouth.

THE ECONOMICS OF INDULGENCE AND RESTRICTION

Here's how much money we spend on indulgence each year:

$3 billion on ice cream
$10 billion on chocolate
$26 billion in vending machines
$86 billion on fast food

And here's how much money we spend restricting ourselves each year:

$3.5 billion on diet soft drinks
$8.8 billion on low-fat and fat-free foods
$11 billion on health foods
$33 billion on weight-loss programs, products, books, and tapes

---

DISORDER OF DESIRE

Like you, I've spent many years trying to free myself from the extremes of deprivation and indulgence. My obsessions with both overeating and undereating helped distract me from feeling painful emotional wounds. I could have spent the rest of my life examining the relationship between my eating habits and my childhood; there was certainly enough to look at. But the past didn't necessarily bear any relationship to what I was eating in the present. When it came to wanting a cheese omelette with french fries, self-examination didn't help much. Like Oscar Wilde, I could "resist anything but temptation." I managed to stay at a reasonable weight, but the struggle was so unpleasant it hardly seemed worth it.

My preoccupation with food eventually became a career. For nine years I helped develop the psychological aspects of the Weight Watchers food plan. My job was to develop techniques and strategies to help overweight people learn self-awareness and self-acceptance as they lost weight.

I scoured the scientific literature searching for clues to the mystery of obesity and why so many proposed solutions have eluded so many intelligent people. Scientists can learn how to duplicate life through cloning; politicians have helped end decades of racial persecution in South Africa. Religious leaders have begun a peace process in the Middle East; astronomers have found signs of life on Mars. Why can't anyone figure out how to help people maintain a healthy weight?

I also spoke with many amazing people, ones who had overcome life-threatening illnesses and unspeakable trage- dies while going to school, managing careers, raising chil- dren, and running households. Yet, when it came to their weight, they were powerless. What accounts for this dispar- ity? Why were they able to endure tremendous sacrifices in their lives but not able to pass up a candy bar? How could they give up bread at Passover, alcohol at Lent, or fast all day during Ramadan, but be unable to resist certain foods?

The Four Noble Truths help us see the answers to these questions: *overeating is a disorder of desire.* Eating problems are the result of not understanding the futility of attachment to desire in a world that is constantly changing. Freedom from eating problems comes from changing your relationship to desire and learning how to make peace with whatever is present. This requires a willingness to explore alternative forms of nourishment that are capable of offering the inner satisfaction that's eluded you for so long.

THE SOUP KITCHEN

One key aspect of the Eightfold Path (Right Action) stresses the importance of generosity. The Buddha said, "If you knew what I do about the power of giving, you wouldn't let a single meal go by without taking the opportunity to give."

So between business trips and helping patients struggle with the burden of abundance, I discovered how emotionally nourishing it was to offer time and resources to a local soup kitchen. At a church meeting hall, free food was provided for between 150 and 200 people. Among them were families who ran out of food stamps and single parents with small children. They gathered for a free hot meal, possibly their only one of the day.

At the soup kitchen, food is a source of delight, not a source of misery. People rarely complain. There are no menus so there are no choices. It's "Take it or leave it." No one turns down food because it is too fattening or sends it back to the kitchen because it wasn't prepared the right way.

Everyone at the soup kitchen receives the same simple meal. Most consist of canned pork and beans or spaghetti and meatballs. Processed turkey loaf with instant mashed potatoes is a special treat. The dining room is small and crowded. It often smells of sweat and dirty clothes. There's an occasional fistfight. People get mad when they are turned down for seconds, and some people get upset when they are told to take their hats off while they eat. Yet there is a palpable feeling of excitement in the dining room, and it's contagious. There's a special feeling of community among those who give and those who receive. For a few moments in the day, people who are normally perceived as outcasts experience a sense of dignity and worthiness that comes from being well fed and treated with kindness. At the same time, people who have the luxury of abundance have the opportunity to help others and share their resources in ways that bring substantial nourishment to both groups.

DIETERS FEED THE HUNGRY

I often left the soup kitchen feeling full and exhilarated. My enthusiasm about the nourishment that comes from helping others led me to start an organization called Dieters Feed the Hungry. The idea was to encourage people struggling with eating problems to expand the ways in which they nourish themselves by practicing generosity and feeding hungry people. I put a small ad in the local newspaper, and the program took off. I matched volunteers and their skills and interests to various soup kitchens and food giveaway programs. Some people made casseroles for battered women's shelters, some people donated eggs to a breakfast program for homeless men, and others served food or washed dishes in local soup kitchens.

I also found out about the need for nutritious food at a prenatal clinic for high-risk pregnancies at a county hospital. A nurse/friend of mine told me that some of the pregnant woman propelled by their own hunger and the hunger of their children had resorted to taking food from the staff refrigerator; others just waited for hours without anything to eat or drink. Volunteers from Dieters Feed the Hungry served hot meals and fresh fruit to the clinic members every week. We also sponsored an infant formula drive. We learned that some of the newborn infants drank soda because their mothers couldn't afford to buy formula or receive the resources from the government-sponsored Women, Infant, Children (WIC) program. Many of the women were drug or alcohol addicted so breast-feeding was not an option. This formula drive generated tremendous community support from individuals and from infant formula providers. Thousands of cases of infant formula were donated to the clinic so that all the mothers had enough formula to feed their infants.

The organization ran by volunteers. All donations went for the purchase of nutritious food. Nevertheless, without spending a penny for publicity, we received a lot of it. Local and national newspaper, magazine, and television reporters ran stories about the nourishing connection between physically feeding others and emotionally nourishing yourself. Our mailing list grew quickly and steadily; many people wanted to start local chapters and groups, and the telephone rang constantly with people from all over the country wanting to know, "How can I get involved? And Where can I help?"

As a result of all the publicity we had received, many key people at Weight Watchers became interested in how they could help hungry people in their local areas. Food drives and local walks were initiated around the country so dieters could feed the hungry.

Just as the organization was taking off and gaining momentum, a firestorm ripped through the Oakland, California, hills and burned down nearly 3,000 houses, including my house and office. Everything was destroyed: the Dieters Feed the Hungry mailing, volunteer, and resource lists, our correspondence, and plans for new projects were burnt to ashes (in addition to everything I owned, except for the shirt on my back).

Not long after the fire, several relatives and dear friends died, including my older brother, my father, my grandmother (who my husband, two brothers, and I had taken care of), and one of my closest friends. Not only was I faced with having to rebuild my life from scratch, I was also faced with tremendous grief. Not surprisingly, I got very sick. I developed pneumonia, a thyroid disorder, and Epstein Barr disease. In order to heal myself, I had to learn to let go of all of my possessions and some of my deepest human connections. I was forced to stop working as the psychological consultant to Weight Watchers and give up developing Dieters Feed the Hungry.

Although Dieters Feed the Hungry is no longer operating, many volunteers have continued to donate their time and resources to the soup kitchens and food giveaway programs they made a commitment to many years ago. They continue to receive a kind of lasting nourishment from giving to others that they can't find in anything they eat. In writing *The Zen of Eating*, I am joining these volunteers and returning to my commitment to giving to others.

I am writing this book as an offering. It's my hope that the insights and changes that come from applying the Four Noble Truths and practicing generosity help transform your emotional hunger into lasting nourishment. I also hope that you will share your physical and emotional resources with hungry people so everyone gets fed and feels nourished, on every level.

The desire crisis that hurts millions of people and helps

almost no one can be transformed. But you're the only one who can make this work. In order to actualize the teachings in this book, you need to practice mindfulness every day for a period of time between thirty and sixty minutes. This commitment to practice helps train the mind to resist chasing desire and return it to the only moment there is. Without that commitment, you can't end emotional hunger and experience the kind of nourishment that lasts. So please, practice mindfulness every day.

No one can practice or apply the wisdom of the Four Noble Truths for you. You are the only one who can experience the power and possibility of these insights and practices. This is why the Buddha insisted, "Do not blindly believe what others say. See for yourself what brings clarity and peace. That is the path for you to follow."

An old Buddhist monk once said, "What boundless joy to know there is no true happiness." He was acknowledging that there is no lasting happiness, just as there is no lasting meal, body weight, or ice cream cone. Things are always changing. That's life. Yet it is possible to find balance in the midst of change and peace in the midst of suffering. But don't believe me, find out for yourself. I hope this book will help you do that.

PART ONE

EMOTIONAL
HUNGER

CHAPTER 1

THERE IS SUFFERING:

Tasting Change

APPLYING THE FIRST NOBLE TRUTH

◎

*What is the Noble Truth of Suffering? Birth is suffering, decay
is suffering, death is suffering; sorrow, lamentation, pain, grief,
and despair are suffering; not to get what one desires is suffering;
in short the five groups of existence are suffering.*

—*THE BUDDHA*

The Buddha made a plain and simple observation about
life that he summed up in the First Noble Truth: *There
is suffering.*

The Sanskrit word for suffering, *dukkha,* literally means *a
wheel off center.* It refers to the empty, uneasy feeling that
lingers as long as you expect something outside yourself to
fulfill you or make you happy. Some call this feeling *emotional hunger.* Others call it *the bottomless pit.* Webster defines
suffering as "the bearing or undergoing of pain, distress, or
injury." The Buddha called all of these things *suffering.*

21

The Buddha didn't say, "There is suffering" because he was a pessimist or because of a difficult childhood. He said, "There is suffering" because he observed that it is impossible to find complete and lasting satisfaction in anything that changes. When you rely on things that change as sources of happiness, there is suffering. This includes, of course, relying on what you weigh and what you eat. You experience an inner emptiness, a feeling of emotional hunger, which comes from expecting satisfaction from things that change.

When you are mindful, you see that things are always changing. For instance, the kind of food you want when you're sick is probably different than the kind you want when you're well. What you eat today is probably going to be different than what you eat tomorrow. But the reality of change is not always easy to remember. We live in a society that often puts out a different message: things last. Just think about how many weight loss plans you've bought into that have promised, "This is the last diet you'll ever need," or how many beauty products that suggest that buying and using them will help make you stay and feel forever young. The pressures to deny suffering and the truth of impermanence are very powerful. When you don't recognize them, they can also be very painful.

INEVITABLE SUFFERING VERSUS OPTIONAL SUFFERING

When you look closely at any type of suffering, you can see that not all suffering is alike. Some suffering is inevitable, and some is optional. This is an important distinction.

Inevitable suffering is a result of changes that are beyond your control. A lot of what's beyond your control has to do with things that are very important to you. Whether you like it or not, your body will change, get sick, and eventually die. Ultimately, you will be separated from the people, the places, and the things that matter most to you. There's nothing you or anyone else can do to prevent these changes from happening; they are part of life. So a certain amount of sadness, loss, and frustration are built in to the framework of being alive. This is inevitable suffering.

Optional suffering is different from inevitable suffering because it is within your control. It comes from your reaction to situations, inevitable or otherwise. Optional suffering is what you add on to whatever happens. It's extra. For example, there may be a certain sadness that comes from the fact that your forty-five-year-old body doesn't look or feel as good as your twenty-five-year-old body. If you have negative opinions about middle-aged bodies (if you think you're over the hill or you're no longer attractive), those opinions are extra, so you take on optional suffering.

KANGAROO MEAT: AGONY OR ECSTASY?

It's easy to notice optional suffering when you look at the way manners, rules of etiquette, and food preferences vary from place to place. What's a norm in one society may seem repulsive in another. What's appropriate to eat is not intrinsic to the food. These judgments are optional, and so is the suffering that comes from them.

An Australian businessman traveled to Paris for the first time. He was shocked and disgusted to find that kangaroo meat was a delicacy in France. To him (and many other Australians), eating kangaroo meat was equivalent to eating rat meat. It sickened him to sit next to someone eating kangaroo meat and listen to him rave about its great flavor. The Australian eventually saw that his discomfort didn't come from watching and listening. It came from his reactions to it, which were rooted in his cultural assumptions about kangaroo meat.

Optional suffering covers a wide range of feelings. You can feel mildly upset that Parisians eat Kangaroo meat or that you've gained so much weight you can't fit into most of your clothes. But it is also possible for your reaction to be much stronger. You may feel deep disgust, hatred, or self-hatred in these situations. Whether your reaction is mild or extreme, all of it is optional suffering. It comes from your reaction, not from anything inevitable.

MENTAL ATTITUDE, SUFFERING, AND HAPPINESS

There's a story about a great Zen master named Won Hyo. It shows the influence of your attitude on optional suffering. As a young man, Won Hyo wanted to understand the truth about human nature, so he set out for the great dry northern plains of China in search of a master. One evening, while crossing the desert, he stopped at a small patch of grass and went to sleep. In the middle of the night, he woke up very thirsty and groped around until he found a container of water. He drank it with great delight and gratitude.

The next morning, Won Hyo woke up and saw that the container was actually a shattered skull, caked with dried blood. His thirst had been quenched by a skull full of bloody rainwater with dead bugs floating in it. Won Hyo felt a huge wave of nausea inside him and then vomited.

But then he experienced a deep realization of the First Noble Truth. He realized that the suffering as well as the happiness he felt came from within. They didn't have anything to do with his direct experience of drinking. They came from his mental attitude toward the experience, not anything that was built in to it. Since reactions come from within, Won Hyo also realized that the option to be happy was just as much of a possibility as the option to suffer.

Here are some examples of a similar dynamic that you'll probably recognize in yourself. Let's say you hate to cook. If only you didn't have to cook, you'd be happy. Cooking takes too much time, nothing turns out well, and no one appreciates all the work involved. But where is the source of suffering? It's within you. You're the one filled with hate and resentment, not the cooking. Cooking is a series of impermanent actions: mixing, stirring, chopping, pouring, squeezing, and shaking. It doesn't have the power to make you happy or miserable. Those reactions are within you. Suffering and happiness come from your mental attitude toward cooking, not from cooking itself. If you don't realize this, you'll spend a lot of time hating cooking unnecessarily. You waste a lot of time and energy focusing on factors that trigger the experience of suffering but are not responsible for them.

Let's look at another example: You love rye bread. You can't wait to buy some fresh rye bread and enjoy it. But when you arrive at the bakery, it's closed. Now the thought of rye bread makes you feel frustrated instead of happy.

Where is the suffering? It's not within the rye bread. There's nothing in the ingredients of rye bread that has the power to make you happy or sad. That power is within you. But if you continue to think that the source of happiness or frustration comes from eating (or not eating) rye bread, you continue searching for happiness where it can't be found, and there is suffering.

THE EXTENT OF INEVITABLE
SUFFERING IS OPTIONAL

There's a beautiful story that illustrates how a change in attitude toward inevitable suffering can change the intensity of it. Even in the worst situation imaginable, some of the suffering may be optional or added on. A grief-stricken mother asked the Buddha to bring her dead child back to life. In response, he asked her to bring him one mustard seed from a house where no one had ever died. The heart-broken woman went door to door in search of a mustard seed. Everyone she met was happy to give her the seed until she explained it must come from a house where no one had died. At that point, each offer of the seed was withdrawn. The woman returned from her search seedless, but with the knowledge that death is universal and part of everyone's life.

This woman's search taught her that no one lives free of loss. She hadn't been singled out for this terrible misfortune, so there was no reason to make things worse by putting up a struggle by feeling so alone and that her pain was unique. Her inevitable suffering wasn't eliminated nor could it be.

But the optional suffering she experienced could be eliminated and it was, once she let go of her struggle against it. The situation wasn't in her control, but her reaction to it was.

OPTIONAL SUFFERING, INNER PEACE, AND MENTAL ATTITUDE

Every challenging situation you encounter offers a similar opportunity. You can learn to minimize the suffering that comes from the struggle over a situation, even though the situation itself is not in your control. This enables you to see an important aspect of the First Noble Truth: The extent of suffering/hunger and inner peace/self-nourishment come from within. Even though a lot of suffering can't be avoided, you can reduce it significantly by learning how to relate to it. You're not bound to your reactions in the way you are bound to your height or to the color of your eyes. In other words, optional suffering offers the possibility of change.

These insights don't come easily. Many of us have a strong and misguided tendency to believe that suffering and happiness come from things outside, rather than inside, ourselves. Under the influence of this misperception, we may respond to certain messages that otherwise would be meaningless if they were understood within the framework of the First Noble Truth. You hope they're true when you hear messages like bananas are possibly the most perfect food in the world, or that certain desserts can be total indulgence and zero guilt. In pursuit of happiness, you continue to chase after things that change, insisting that there must be something that works: a diet, a flavor of ice cream, or whatever. You keep trying to find *something* that works.

HOW CAN YOU EAT AT A TIME LIKE THIS?

If you can't see your struggle or identify your reactions, even more suffering gets generated. You stay stuck in the endless suffering/hunger cycle and often drag others into it with you. So the suffering/hunger cycle keeps growing. Consider this example.

Joyce and her mother-in-law accompanied Joyce's husband, Henry, to the hospital where he was to have knee surgery. The operation and recovery time would be about two hours, and then Henry would be ready to go home. After seeing Henry settled and wishing him well, Joyce and her mother-in-law went to the waiting room. Joyce suggested getting something to eat. Her mother-in-law snapped back, "How can you eat at a time like this?" She was angry (and full of optional suffering) because Joyce was focusing on food instead of her son. In her eyes, "eating at a time like this" was a sign of insensitivity.

Eating "at a time like this" is neither right nor wrong; they are different responses to the same situation. From the point of view of the mother-in-law, Joyce was wrong and she was right. She was blinded by suffering and added to it by confusing her reaction with the situation that triggered it. She didn't understand her role in the situation.

On the other hand, Joyce was able to acknowledge suffering and choose how to respond to it. She saw eating "at a time like this" as a practical and enjoyable way to pass the time. It didn't have anything to do with her devotion to her husband. She felt mildly insulted that her mother-in-law saw the situation in a different way, but Joyce also realized she had options. She could get angry with her mother-in-law for implying that she wasn't a good wife and create more optional suffering, or she could remind herself that insult and anger come from within her, and not from the situation itself. Joyce recognized her vulnerability to these feelings, but she didn't act it out. She decided not to escalate the suffering by adding anything to it.

Once you're stuck in reacting, there's no end to the suffering/hunger you can experience. There are always people or situations to blame that keep suffering/hunger alive. If you don't realize that the source is within you, you keep trying to fill the emotional vacuum. Until you see the relationship between mental attitude and suffering, you continue to search for satisfaction everywhere and find it nowhere.

GETTING OUT OF THE SUFFERING/HUNGER TRAP

To end the destructive cycle of escalating suffering, you need to identify your suffering in the first place. In other words, you have to be able to see suffering in order to be free of it. Suffering has many different facets to it. Take a look at some of the types of suffering that occur and notice the ones that are most familiar to you:

- **Ordinary suffering**: feeling deprived no matter how much or what you eat

- **Emotional suffering**: feeling powerless around appealing food and anxious about your ability to limit what you eat, feeling embarrassed about your body, beating yourself up for falling into the same eating patterns over and over again, obsessing about what to eat

- **Social suffering**: feeling second class because of your body size, avoiding certain events because you're uncomfortable in your clothes

- **Financial suffering**: overspending on diet food, tapes, books, and programs that don't work; feeling ripped off

- **Physical suffering**: Feeling heavy, lethargic, and uncomfortable

REMEMBER: THINGS CHANGE

It's crucial to recognize that you are not eternally over-weight—nor any particular weight. Nor are you eternally hungry or full. These situations, no matter how compelling they seem to be in the moment, are fleeting. While you can't wish them away, you do have control over how you respond to them. You can respond to your hunger by gorging yourself on everything in sight, or you can observe the urge to eat, and know with full confidence that it won't last.

You can despair over a number on the scale, or you can remind yourself that weight, like everything else, changes. You don't have to remain a victim of circumstance. You can take responsibility for your reactions. Since things are always changing, there are always choices you can make. But you need to make the effort, especially when you feel drawn to advertising messages that suggest that if you buy this or eat that, you'll never feel deprived or be inconvenienced. Nothing has the power to do that.

BE MINDFUL OF CHANGE

When you are mindful, you realize that change is part of everything. Everything from your current weight and eating habits to your favorite restaurant to your most preferred kitchen gadget all share the same destiny. They will change at some time or another. Change is just as much a part of pleasant experiences as it is of painful ones. Good feelings come and go, just as bad feelings do. Delicious meals end just as lousy ones do. Fullness changes to hunger, and if you're lucky, hunger becomes fullness again. Your body weight shifts from day to day, month to month, year to year, and decade to decade, whether you want it to or not. Passions for particular foods change. Your favorite meal as a child is probably different from what you loved most as a teenager, and that's probably different from your favorite meal today.

By paying even closer attention, you can see change on more and more refined levels. For instance, what you call eating breakfast is one aspect of an ongoing series of changes. The toast began in the wheat fields and then processing plants before it became bread on the grocery store shelf and eventually to your toaster. As soon as you take the first bite of toast, breakfast has changed on many different levels.

APPRECIATING THE MOMENT

When you know that nothing lasts, you can appreciate eating in a new way. You can see for yourself why the Buddha said, "Life is filled with suffering. But it also contains many wonders. Being in touch with both is to truly encounter life, to see it deeply."

When you pay attention to what's in front of you, there's no need to look for satisfaction elsewhere. What you're looking for is right in front of you. Instead of complaining about the same old steamed vegetables, you can marvel at their many characteristics: texture, color, temperature, shape, and size. When you feel impatient to drink your morning coffee, you can listen to the multitone gurgles of the coffeemaker. No matter how often you hear them, each gurgle is unique. It will never be duplicated. Neither will anything else.

As you become mindful of the many wonders in life, mundane tasks like fixing a bag lunch can be transformed into a cornucopia of delight. You are present enough to enjoy the graceful motion of each swipe of mustard on the bread and notice the colors of everything involved: brown bread, yellow mustard, green lettuce, purple onion, red tomato, and pale-white cheese. The variety of colors and motions is a lot more fun than wanting the dull task to be over.

WAYS TO BECOME MINDFUL OF THE FIRST NOBLE TRUTH

1. Notice the ways you suffer over what you weigh and how you look. Then ask yourself, "How much of this suffering is inevitable? How much of it is optional?"

2. Notice impermanence throughout the day. Watch how meals, thoughts, tastes, and feelings all come and go. Can you find anything that remains exactly the same? How does seeing impermanence change your relationship to what you eat and how you feel about yourself?

3. Notice what triggers the feeling of suffering/hunger within you. Who are the people and what are the situations that trigger these feelings?

4. Think about what it would mean to eat your next meal as if this was the first or the last time. It's true that every meal is your first meal because it's unique and will never be here again. It's also true that your next meal could be your last meal. Knowing this, what would you do differently throughout the meal? Would you be more likely to complain or to savor every bite?

5. Distinguish between a painful experience and your reaction to it. For instance, if your pants feel too tight, you may react in a number of different ways: sometimes you

laugh, other times you cry, and other times you turn against yourself by overeating. Do you tend to believe the reaction comes from the situation or from you?

Consider these examples:

- You feel empty but don't know why.
- You get excited about the latest celebrity weight-loss cure.
- You hate what was served for dinner.

6. Label your reactions just as you would greet someone you know by name. This will help you realize the difference between your reactions to a situation and the situation itself.

For example, if you:

- Are bored with oatmeal, notice *boredom*.
- Are angry at your family, notice *anger*.
- Can't figure out what to eat, notice *indecision*.
- Eat everything in sight, notice *out of control*.
- Are embarrassed by your body, notice *embarrassment*.

Then remind yourself, *"These reactions are within me. They're not built into the situation."*

CHAPTER 2

ATTACHMENT TO DESIRE CAUSES SUFFERING:

A Change of Heart Helps Change the Mind

APPLYING THE SECOND NOBLE TRUTH

◎

What, now, is the Noble Truth of the Origin of Suffering? It is craving, which gives rise to fresh rebirth, and, bound up with pleasure and lust, now here, now there, finds ever-fresh delight. But where does this craving arise and take root? Wherever in the world there are delightful and pleasurable things, there this craving arises and takes root.

—*THE BUDDHA*

The Buddha doesn't just say, "Suffering is a fact," and leave it at that. He gets to the root of suffering and points to the cause of it. In the Second Noble Truth, he states that attachment to desire causes suffering.

Notice that the Second Noble Truth does not say *desire* causes suffering. It says *attachment* to desire causes suffering. It's the "I've got to (need to, have to, want to, love to, hate to, don't want to)" part that causes suffering, not the desire itself.

HEADS AND TAILS

Sometimes the desire for happiness is compared to the head of a snake, and the desire to avoid unhappiness is compared to the tail. If you grasp the head, the snake will bite you. If you grasp the tail, the snake will also bite you because the head and tail both belong to the same snake. No matter which end you grasp, the results are the same. You suffer.

Attachment to desire, also described as *clinging* or *grasping*, means you are so absorbed in your desire that you can't see clearly. You respond as if you operated on automatic pilot: buy this, eat that, wear this, don't weigh that. You see only what you're lusting after, like a handful of cashews or a pint of your favorite ice cream, but you don't see the force behind it. This is called getting lost or being blinded by desire. What you want feels like a requirement, not an option. The Second Noble Truth invites you to examine the relationship between grasping desires and suffering so you can see how this relationship works for yourself.

Take the desire to eat. It happens many times a day.

Sometimes the desire is quite mellow. You can decide to eat or not, depending on the situation. Other times, the desire to eat feels like a powerful engine is driving you forward at breakneck speed. That engine is your attachment to eating. It's screaming, "I want something to eat and I want it *now*."

THE NATURE OF DESIRE

Desires pull like magnets, and they don't discriminate. When it comes to desire, there is no code of ethics that tells you to grasp only what's helpful and not hurtful to yourself or others. You can see this at the grocery store when you're hungry and filled with the desire to eat. Everything looks tantalizing. Even things you might normally not be attracted to, like a can of premade frosting, look appealing. Another time, when you're not hungry, not in that heightened state of desire, it's hard to believe you lusted after something you don't even like. That's the power of desire.

Desires are also deceptive. You are fooled into believing that satisfying them will bring you happiness. That's their allure; it's how they capture your attention. But what you desire often leads you down a dead-end alley. There's no lasting happiness to be found in any desire because what we want changes. Things that change are unreliable, so investing in them is unwise.

It's difficult to remember the Wisdom of the First Noble Truth when a huge wave of desire overcomes you. When it strikes, the desire for a brownie feels terribly compelling. The desire to find the perfect wine to complement a meal feels extremely urgent. But these aren't the keys to happiness, and they certainly aren't the keys to lasting nourishment. These are *empty waves of desire*, rising and passing away. That's the lesson of the Second Noble Truth. But these are insights you must discover for yourself over and over again.

You may be wondering, "What's wrong with desire?" In fact, nothing is *wrong* with desire. Desires are a normal and healthy part of life. Asking for chicken soup when you're sick with a cold or looking forward to a romantic meal on Valentine's Day is perfectly natural. Wanting to share restaurant recommendations or recipes with friends is fun. The desire to teach your children good table manners and set limits on sweets is laudable, even if it's an uphill battle.

Yet, if every desire were satisfied continuously, one after the other, for the rest of your life, you'd still want more. That's the nature of desire. It *wants*. The number and variety of things to get, have, buy, or be is endless. This allows for endless opportunities to suffer.

HUNGRY GHOSTS

There's a powerful image to depict the futility of pursuing one object of desire after another: the Hungry Ghost. Hungry Ghosts are large, mythic beings with huge, distended bellies and extremely narrow throats. They try to eat, but their narrow throats prevent them from getting the fulfillment they crave. No matter what they do and how hard they try, they feel empty and unsatisfied. The Hungry Ghost is not just a figure in Buddhist mythology. There's a Hungry Ghost in each of us, too.

Every time you pursue your desires blindly, you activate

the Hungry Ghost. It often takes the form of a convincing inner voice that says, "You can feel satisfied all the time. You can make the good times last. Keep looking. *It's out there.*" You believe this voice, so you get more cookies, try another restaurant, enroll in the latest get-thin-quick program, or whatever else you believe can satisfy you. But it's never enough.

The more you respond to your Hungry Ghost, the more demanding it becomes. It hammers away at you, spitting out desire after desire: eat more grains, eat less fat, enroll in a cooking school, get a new blade for the blender, buy another vitamin, join a gym. You're so busy chasing desire after desire that you don't see that the Hungry Ghost is running your life. It creates trap after trap. If you don't recognize the presence of the Hungry Ghost, you wonder why you feel so bad when all these things and experiences are supposed to make you feel so good.

ONE DESIRE AFTER ANOTHER

Katie is a divorced social worker. In many ways she's well off. She has family money and two well-educated and hard-working daughters. But Katie is obsessed with food and losing weight. In other words, her Hungry Ghost is in charge. Because Katie doesn't recognize its demanding presence, she responds to the Hungry Ghost as if she were an intimidated employee determined to please a tyrannical boss. She eats bags of cookies and cartons of ice cream and then signs up for the latest weight-loss scheme (the all-sweets diet, the new mail-order mineral diet). Or she devours boxes of candy and then buys all the new low-fat cookbooks. But whatever she tries or gets is never enough. Her Hungry Ghost makes sure of that.

DRY DRUNKS

The Hungry Ghost has a cousin, the Dry Drunk. (There's no specific reference to the Dry Drunk in Buddhist texts, but the idea behind it is there.) Instead of trying to compulsively fulfill one desire after another, Dry Drunks compulsively want to control their desires through abstinence or substitution. Instead of attachment to more and more, the Dry Drunk is fanatically attached to self-deprivation or to different kinds of attachments. The Dry Drunk mentality is similar to that of the Hungry Ghost. The feelings are extreme because the level of attachment is so strong.

A Dry Drunk previously hooked on sugar, for instance, now avoids sugar altogether. On the surface, it looks like the desire for sugar has been eliminated, but in fact, the desire for sugar is as strong as ever. That desire says, "I still want sugar. Give me sugar." The Dry Drunk responds by saying, "Shut up and be quiet. No more sugar for you!" The combination of demanding self-deprivation and unacknowledged attachment is often the perfect setup for binge eating. The Hungry Ghost demands sugar because it's what the Dry Drunk insists it can't have. No matter who wins the battle, there are no winners. If there's a binge, the Hungry Ghost gets reinforced to want more and more. If there's no binge, there's usually some kind of desire substitution. Now the Dry Drunk eats only sugar-free foods, like sugar-free ice cream, candy, soda, and gum. But this is no permanent solution. The source of the problem—the attachment to desire—is still in the driver's seat, so there's still suffering.

GETTING TO THE ROOT OF DESIRE

Keep in mind that the Buddha was a realist. He said, "Recognize desire, and see it clearly. You need to learn about desire and how it works." There are three types of desire, all related to each other:

1. *Sense desires.* These desires demand that you satisfy the five senses: seeing, touching, tasting, feeling, and smelling. You crave the pleasure these senses offer; the more the better. If one cookie tastes good, two would be even more satisfying.

2. *Avoidance desires.* This is the desire to get rid of what's unpleasant. You pull away from things that cause pain or discomfort. You want to get rid of your potbelly, thunder thighs, thick waist, or flabby arms once and for all.

3. *Becoming desires.* With these desires, you want what's missing. You experience a feeling of inner emptiness that you want to fill up, so you want something new like a digital scale or another kind of teakettle that doesn't make so much noise.

Once you've learned to identify your desires, the next step is to identify your attachment to them. Attachments are often compared to the roots of a tree. You can cut down a tree thousands of times, but if the roots remain strong and healthy, the tree will still grow back. In other words, no matter how many times desires get satisfied, new desires pop up to replace the old ones. Similarly, you can cut back a desire, like wanting chocolate, but if the attachment at the root of the desire is healthy and firmly planted, one desire will be substituted for another. The Dry Drunk will find alternative desires and become attached to those. For instance, the Dry Drunk will convince you to eat jelly beans instead of chocolate, carrots instead of cashews, English muffins instead of bagels.

It's easy to confuse attachment to desire with the object of it. The common tendency is to pay attention to what you want. But this is a trap. What you want is endless. It's the Hungry Ghost that can never feel satisfied. You need to see the Hungry Ghost but not get distracted by what it wants.

Here are some examples of how to distinguish attachment to desire from the object of it.

ATTACHMENT	OBJECT OF DESIRE
I want to	lose weight.
I need to	keep off the weight I lost.
I can't stand	how much money I waste on junk food.
I love	romantic, candlelight dinners.
I'm terrified of	parties where there is a lot of tempting food.

Let's look at the first example: *I want to lose weight.* This desire to lose weight is not a problem in and of itself. If there's an attachment to the desire to lose weight, the rest of story is predictable. The Hungry Ghost keeps searching for the perfect diet or the perfect body weight and then never feels satisfied. It always wants more. In other words, whatever you do eventually stops working and you're back to square one again.

The key is to see that "I want to" (the attachment desire) and "lose weight" (the object of the desire) are two very different beasts. Although it may feel as though these two are inextricably combined, they are not. Suffering doesn't come from the object "to lose weight." "To lose weight" is neutral. It has no power, and it feels no pain. Suffering comes from the feeling of wanting. This *wanting* is what hurts, not your weight. Suffering is caused by your wanting, and wanting is your attachment to desire.

The experience of wanting is to *want*, and what you want changes ceaselessly. What's more, the number of objects to want are limitless. If the object *to lose weight* wasn't there, the Hungry Ghost within would want something else. The Hungry Ghost has no loyalty to what it wants, it just wants one thing after another.

PARTIES

Let's take a look at the last example from above: *I'm terrified of parties where there is a lot of tempting food.* When you're attached to feeling terrified of parties, you avoid parties because you don't want to be tempted by the food. You worry about receiving invitations to parties, especially around holidays. Just one party could ruin a week's worth of weight-loss efforts.

When you see your state of mind clearly, you recognize that the energy you spend being terrified of parties is misguided. This pain doesn't come from a party; parties don't cause pain. Suffering comes from *the experience of being terrified* and *wanting to avoid* parties. If you weren't terrified of parties, terror would find something else to fear. *Feeling terrified* is an attachment to desire on the lookout for an object to be terrified of. It doesn't matter what the object is; terror doesn't care.

The *feeling* of terror within you is what needs your attention, not another object to distract your attention from it. When you focus on the feeling of terror, it loosens the grip on the object, in this case, parties. Once you identify your attachment to desire as separate from the object of it, you isolate the source of suffering so you can begin to address it.

The ability to separate attachments from objects of desire is an ongoing challenge. The Hungry Ghost works hard to keep you searching for things to satisfy the chronic hunger for more. You must work even harder to pay attention to what's fueling this search instead of participating in it.

GRASPING ATTACHMENTS HURTS, PREFERENCES DO NOT

Preferences aren't destined to create suffering. Only *grasping* at preferences has the power to do that. For instance, if you'd rather be two sizes smaller, that preference is no problem. But if you're really attached to wanting to be a smaller size, that attachment can create problems. You may feel driven to take extreme measures like using diet pills or trying a crash diet that's nutritionally unsound. Or you may beat yourself up to such a degree that you become depressed and withdrawn. In other words, attachments can be dangerous and create a lot of suffering.

Strong attachments, not preferences, have the potential to trigger your own suffering, and they have the potential to hurt others as well. Carol dated a man who enjoyed dining out. While eating a roast chicken dinner together, Carol chewed on the chicken bones and ate the skin on the baked potato. This was the part of the meal she truly savored. She noticed her date left the chicken bones to the side of his plate and carefully separated the inside of the potato from the skin. When she casually remarked on this difference between them, he responded, "I learned that chewing on bones was tacky and eating potato skins was something only peasants do."

Carol felt that her date was sharing more than just an innocent preference. His attachment to his opinion revealed a bias that she found insulting. Her date didn't apologize because he believed he was entitled to his opinion. It was his attachment to the opinion that bothered Carol, more than the opinion itself. Their relationship ended that evening. Carol eventually married a man with his own set of preferences, but he didn't express them by being judgmental or self-righteous. Of course, each member of the couple had their differences, but they were careful to not confuse their preferences with their attachment to them.

IDENTITY

The suffering generated from our attachments really heats up when we build an identity around them. For instance, at times we define ourselves by certain preferences: "I'm a chocolate lover;" "I'm an Italian food freak;" "I'm a deli devotee;" or I'm an Indian food snob." Once you establish an identity around something, there's pressure to support and defend it. That's a form of suffering in and of itself. Defending an identity takes time and energy. As a restaurant buff, you only want to go to the places where you get the best burritos or the flakiest croissants; you need to avoid the second-rate places.

Your identification with something can be so strong, you lose perspective on what's really true: you are not your attachments. There are many different pieces that make up *you* and these pieces are always changing. In the morning you may start out as Mom or Dad. But that identity is always changing. In Buddhist psychology, there's no real *you*. That's a concept that describes many interrelated facets of experiences. But when you're strongly identified with one of these facets, it feels like you are your attachments, and this creates suffering.

Attachment to Real Bagels

Dan, an ex–New Yorker, is identified with being an authority on bagels. He's always complaining that there are no decent bagels where he lives. He's quick to explain what he believes are the critical distinctions between steamed, boiled, and wood-fired bagels. It upsets him when anyone stands up for the quality of local bagels, especially the ones with chocolate chips. His temper flares up. "Those are not *real* bagels," he insists. "They're an insult! I know what a real bagel tastes like!" He is so attached to his identity as a bagel expert that he feels he has no choice but to argue with friends who disagree with him. Everyone suffers. Dan feels frustrated when he's not recognized as right. His friends don't like being yelled at and made to feel like their opinions are second-rate.

Lobster Bisque

Julie calls herself a "foodie." This is her self-proclaimed identity. She knows a lot about food: what's best, what's in season, what's hot, and what's not. She also knows where to order the best of everything. She takes pride in knowing all this information and especially likes sharing it with friends who depend on her advice. It makes her feel in the know.

On a balmy summer evening, Julie and some friends ate in one of Julie's favorite restaurants. It was jammed. Nothing that Julie ordered was available. At one point, she was unable to tolerate it anymore. She found herself jumping up and screaming at the waiter, "Do you know how long I've been waiting to eat your lobster bisque? What kind of restaurant runs out of its most famous dish?" Immediately after the outburst, Julie was overcome by shame and embarrassment. Her desire for a lovely evening with friends and her reputation as a sophisticated restaurant connoisseur were both shot. Her attachment to her identity as a person who knows where to find the best of everything created suffering, but it also taught her an important lesson: feeling compelled to defend an identity can be very painful.

The suffering that is created often spreads out in a ripple effect. Not only do you hurt yourself when there's grasping, others get hurt as well. Julie's attachment to being a "foodie" and Dan's attachment to being an authority on bagels had an unpleasant impact on many people. But sometimes attachments can have even a stronger and more serious effect as the next story shows.

NASRUDIN'S EGGPLANT

Nasrudin is a legendary character in Turkish folklore. He is often used to illustrate the antics of the human mind because he can be silly, clever, and mystical all at once. Nasrudin and a friend once went to a restaurant and decided to share a plate of eggplant. They argued fiercely as to whether the eggplant should be stuffed or fried. Each was attached to his identity about the best way to prepare and enjoy eggplant. Tired and hungry, Nasrudin yielded to his friend's wish to order it stuffed. His companion suddenly collapsed off his chair and onto the floor. Nasrudin jumped out of his seat.

"Are you going for a doctor?" asked someone at the next table.

"No, you fool," shouted Nasrudin. "I'm going to see whether it's too late to change the order."

Nasrudin was so attached to the kind of eggplant he wanted, he saw the accident as an opportunity to satisfy his desire rather than help his friend. Attachments to identity can narrow the perspective to such a degree, they overshadow someone's need for help, put friendships in jeopardy, or trigger the end of a relationship.

IDENTITY CRISES

Dotty identifies herself as someone with total recall of the food served at every event she'd been to in the past thirty years. She says things like, "Oh, Sally's wedding in 1981—the worst roast beef I've ever had. It was dry as a bone and overdone." Dotty also identifies her friends by their relationship to food. She once introduced a neighbor by saying, "This is my friend Rita. She's a great baker, but she can't fry an egg." Rita was insulted and refused to speak to Dotty for a month. Rita thought she was a good cook in every way. That's the identity she was attached to, and she resented the one that Dotty assigned to her. Like Nasrudin, Rita and Dotty were blinded by their attachments to certain identities. The tension between them as a result of this identity crisis was costly. The two women never felt the same about each other since that incident. But strong attachments to identity (assigned to yourself or to others) can have an even stronger impact and trigger the end of a friendship.

ATTACHMENT TO WHAT'S ENOUGH

When Elizabeth and Deena decided to hold a wedding shower for a mutual friend, they were surprised to find out how different their views were on what was enough food. Planning what to serve created a lot of friction between them. To Elizabeth, enough meant having the exact amount of food for each guest so nothing would be wasted. To Deena, enough meant everyone could have as much as they want (or more) and take leftovers home. Each was strongly attached to her own identity and highly critical of the other. Deena thought Elizabeth was cheap. Elizabeth thought Deena was extravagant. They couldn't reach a compromise until another person intervened. The upshot was that Deena brought a little less food than she would have; Elizabeth brought a little more. But the incident ended their fourteen years of friendship. Deena didn't want to be friends with someone who she believed didn't have the spirit of generosity; Elizabeth didn't want to be friends with someone she believed didn't care about wasting food.

All of these examples show how strong attachments to identity can create a lot of pain and suffering. When you become so preoccupied with wanting what you want or hating what you hate because of who you think you are, the potential to create suffering keeps growing and can even be life threatening.

MARTIN'S COOKING

Martin is a busy working parent. Martin loves preparing food for the week and usually spends Sundays creating new batches of spaghetti sauce, a few roasted chickens, and, if there's time, a casserole or two. Martin says he feels possessed by cooking, as if he had been given a drug injection. He gets so absorbed with wanting to make the sauce really outstanding or trying a new chicken recipe that he goes into an altered state. In other words, he becomes so totally blinded by desire that he sees nothing else but that desire. Like Nasrudin, who was blinded by the desire to eat a certain kind of eggplant, Martin was blinded by the desire to cook different kinds of food.

One Sunday afternoon, while Martin was in one of these desire trances, he scrambled around the kitchen tasting sauce, stirring noodles, and checking quantities in the three cookbooks he had open on the counter. It wasn't until a neighbor appeared at the door with his three-year-old daughter that he realized the child had left the kitchen and wandered out of the house. The spell of desire suddenly broke. Martin was mortified that he could lose himself so completely in his desire for cooking that he lost track of his daughter. That event and the tragic consequences that could have come from it served as a wake-up call. Martin realized that his attachment to cooking was dangerous and decided not to cook when he was solely responsible for his daughter.

When you're so identified with grasping and there's no awareness of it, suffering can spread like wildfire. Next time you're in a buffet or a cafeteria line, notice how some people behave. They're so driven by the desire to eat that they push and grab at food as if this were going to be their last meal. It can be very unpleasant and create suffering, especially if people fear there won't be enough food or enough of their favorite food.

The same kind of attachments that you see acted out in a buffet line also get acted out on a much larger scale. The attachment to fear about getting enough is part of the reason why there are wars, famine, nuclear weapons, and murder. These events all grow out of grasping desires and generate layers of suffering that can last for generations. While you alone may not have the power to prevent or stop any of these destructive events, you can take responsibility for learning about your own attachments and the suffering those attachments create within you and for others. The willingness to make peace with these attachments in order to end the suffering they create is the foundation for your inner peace, and it's also the foundation for peace between friends, within families and communities, and ultimately, within the entire world.

WAYS TO BECOME MORE MINDFUL OF THE SECOND NOBLE TRUTH

1. Learn about desire and your relationship to it.

• Is there a specific body weight you need to be to feel good about yourself?

• What food habits and table manners are you attached to?

• Have these attachments created suffering in your life?

2. Recognize the Hungry Ghost and how it works.

• Listen for the Hungry Ghost, and give it a name.

• How would you describe it? As desperate? Sneaky? Demanding? Hurting?

• What does the Hungry Ghost try to get you to buy, do, get, become, own, or get rid of?

• In what situations does the Hungry Ghost appear the most?

3. Take stock of suffering. Think about how much suffering you have created for yourself and for others by your attachment to:

- Eating habits and manners
- Certain food preferences
- Fear about getting enough
- Wanting to weigh less and/or look different

4. Take stock of what you know about the Second Noble Truth. What experiences have you had that help you realize the wisdom of the following statements?

- You can't end suffering without awareness of your attachments.
- No matter how many times attachment gets the object, it's never enough.
- Desires are just thoughts in your mind and feelings in your body.
- *You* and *your desire* are not the same.
- Desires can disappear as suddenly as they appear.

PART TWO

THE END OF EMOTIONAL HUNGER

CHAPTER 3

SUFFERING ENDS BY LETTING GO OF ATTACHMENT TO DESIRE:

Learning to Let Things Be

APPLYING THE THIRD NOBLE TRUTH

◎

*What is the Noble Truth of the end of suffering? It is the
complete fading away and extinction of this attachment
(craving), its forsaking and abandonment, liberation and
detachment from it. The extinction of wanting more, the extinction
of wanting less, the extinction of not seeing things clearly: this is
called freedom, or the end of suffering.*

—*THE BUDDHA*

The Third Noble Truth presents the solution to the
problem and cause of emotional hunger. It states: Suffering ends by letting go of attachment to desire. Letting

go of suffering is a process. It involves learning how to dissolve the source of suffering that drives you to eat but never feel satisfied. You let go of the "I've *got to (need to, have to, love to, hate to, want to, don't want to)*" feelings that lie at the heart of suffering/emotional hunger, and that bond you to the objects of desire (lose weight, eat more cookies, exercise, etc.). When there's no grasping, there's a spacious feeling of acceptance with the way things are. It's this experience that offers the nourishment you've been looking for.

Letting go *doesn't* mean annihilating, rejecting feelings, or pretending that you don't have strong feelings. There's no point in saying, "I'm not into losing weight, I've let go of that," when you're really lusting after a slim body. It's equally absurd to deny being angry when you're so enraged that you can hardly contain yourself. This is fooling yourself, not letting go. Letting go means learning how to become intimate with the lust and rage and learning how to relate to these attachments without grasping, acting out, or repressing them. This is a lifelong task that takes a lot of practice, patience, and compassion for yourself.

MARILYN'S PATTERN OF REJECTION AND LETTING GO OF IT

Marilyn, a clothing designer in her late thirties, wanted to reshape her eating habits because she had gained a lot of weight. Very few of her elegant clothes fit her anymore. During the process of losing weight, Marilyn regularly had images about being rejected. When she was nine, Marilyn was rejected by a school friend and was distraught about it for months. She was an only child and he was her only friend. Marilyn depended on walking to school with him and playing together on weekends. She concluded that there was something bad about her that caused her only friend to leave. Her rational mind kept saying, "It's ridiculous to be upset about something that happened so long ago," but her behavior told a different story. She was driven by the fear of rejection and that fear had become an integral part of her self-image. Marilyn was terrified of people leaving her. She anticipated rejection wherever she went. She ate and overate to compensate for intense feelings of loneliness.

Marilyn decided to pay attention to how this childhood experience was impacting her adult life. That decision initiated her into the letting-go process. It's hard to let go unless you know what you need to let go of. Letting go for Marilyn meant learning to become intimate with the fear of rejection: how she anticipated rejection and even initiated it, both with others and within herself.

Marilyn observed these patterns the way she would watch an actress on a movie screen. This offered her a sense of detachment so that she could be more objective about what she was seeing.

Marilyn began noticing many things: her aloof attitude, her preference to stay uninvolved, the amount of time she spent worrying about being rejected, anticipating how much it was going to hurt, and the feelings of relief when she was alone.

Rather than getting upset or frustrated by what she observed, Marilyn acknowledged the presence of these feelings. She watched them and realized that they all changed at one point or another. She was surprised to find that the more familiar she became with feeling rejected, the more open she was to others, and the more others opened to her. Her relationship to food also changed. The more she allowed those feelings to come and go, the less she needed to cut off that process by overeating.

Investigating her relationship to rejection was the doorway to freedom. In other words, Marilyn let go of her fear of rejection through her willingness to experience all the facets of that fear without grasping or clinging. She realized how much suffering she had perpetuated within herself by avoiding those feelings. When she felt these feelings instead of rejecting them, she was no longer re-creating the conditions for rejection that were based on her early childhood experience.

LETTING GO IS LETTING BE

The key to letting go of attachment to desire is to acknowledge and feel the experiences of grasping and clinging within you. This isn't easy. If you don't like the feeling of rejection, there's grasping. You want to get rid of rejection. As Marilyn learned, rejecting rejection only intensified the fear of it, her loneliness, and her habit of overeating.

There's nothing inherently wrong with fear or hatred or even aggression. But when you're attached to them and take them personally or act them out mindlessly, you create suffering by cutting off the nourishment supply they offer. It's impossible to connect with your own vulnerability, compassion, and gentleness when you're caught up in hating yourself or wanting to be right in an argument or having to be the best cook in town.

Marilyn realized that her painful pattern of behavior was related to early experiences of rejection, but that understanding wasn't enough to end the suffering. Letting go is not an intellectual exercise to see how smart you are. You can come up with all the rational reasons in the world to explain away attachments to desire, but if you don't actually let go of them, they'll continue to be a source of suffering.

By staying with the raw feelings of grasping (hatred, love, self-righteousness, boredom, or whatever) you open up to awareness itself. Your willingness to stay with these feelings transcends your attachment to them because in the moment of awareness, those concepts disappear. There's not even a you there; there's just acceptance. When your mind is free from attachments to desire, it assumes a natural state of balance and a spacious feeling of nourishment. The deep nourishment that comes from letting go serves as lasting food for your mind and heart.

This creates space for new possibilities and choices that otherwise would not be available. You can still have a strong desire to lose weight, but when you're not attached to that desire, you also have the freedom to choose how to respond to it. You don't feel compelled to latch on to the latest weight-loss gimmick or meal replacement bar. You can make a reasonable decision about the best way to go about it, depending on the circumstances of your life and what you know about yourself.

In fact, Marilyn continued to experience fear of rejection, but it no longer had the grip that it once had on her. She was familiar with the many facets of it. When these feelings came up within her, she allowed them to arise and pass away without interference. They didn't cut her off from opportunities to enjoy herself, like going to parties or taking walks with friends.

You can practice letting go of anything: feeling deprived, beliefs about your self-image, the desire to be thin, wanting dessert every day, or needing to feel desirable at the expense of your self-respect. Letting go of an *attachment to hatred* is no different than letting go of *an attachment to love.* Letting go of *attachment to anything* allows a spacious feeling of peace to expand and breathe within you.

Letting go doesn't mean any of these desires disappear. It means that they no longer have control over you. Your response to them changes from feelings of a requirement, to realizing there are options. You can be lonely and not overeat. You can feel anxious without judging yourself. You can be a bagel expert or have strong opinions about proper table manners and eating habits and not create suffering for yourself or others. In short, you are no longer a slave to your desires, to your Hungry Ghost or to that inner authority that's constantly telling you to look for happiness where it can't be found. Above all, you don't have to be beholden to patterns of behavior that don't serve you well.

NASRUDIN'S NEIGHBOR

Nasrudin was eating a simple meal of chickpeas and bread at the same time his neighbor was dining on a sumptuous meal provided by the emperor. His neighbor suggested, "If you would learn to flatter the emperor, then you wouldn't have to eat chickpeas and bread." Nasrudin replied, "If you would learn to let go of those sumptuous meals and live on chickpeas and bread, then you wouldn't have to flatter the emperor."

Nasrudin and his neighbor had different relationships toward eating well. His neighbor was attached to eating well. He needed to eat a certain kind of meal in order to be happy with it. But his need to eat a certain way meant he was beholden to his desires. He wasn't free to enjoy a simple meal; he needed sumptuous ones. He was compelled to flatter the emperor; he wasn't free to behave in a more authentic way.

On the other hand, Nasrudin wasn't attached to eating well. He had let go of it. Nasrudin could enjoy the simplicity of his meal and didn't have to flatter anyone. Unlike his friend, Nasrudin could preserve his dignity instead of compromising it. He wasn't beholden to a pattern of behavior that didn't serve him well or that created a sense of suffering within him. He didn't need sumptuous meals to support an image of himself in this way. He was free of that.

A CLOSER LOOK AT LETTING GO

Let's look at a familiar experience and go through the process step by step. Let's say you want to let go of mindless eating. You hate feeling that you can't eat whatever you want, whenever you want it. It makes you feel deprived. Here's what to do:

Step One: Identify the cause of suffering (the attachment to desire). The feeling of hatred is your attachment to the desire to eat mindlessly. It's what binds you to this desire and causes suffering. That feeling of hatred is the focus of the letting-go process.

Step Two: Explore how the attachment feels within you.
Make the effort to become familiar with hatred. What's it
like to hate? Where do you feel hatred in your body? What
thoughts do you have about it in your mind? Is it comfortable or painful to hate?

*Step Three: Explore your relationship to the attach-
ment.* Learn about how you relate to the attachment.
This is what binds you to it and keeps the suffering alive.
Do you like or dislike the feeling of hatred? Do you want
it to stay or do you want to make it go away? If you
don't like the feeling of hatred, there's usually resistance
to feeling it. Resistance to hatred uncovers another layer
of attachment, another source of suffering. There's hatred
toward mindless eating (your attachment) and there's also
a feeling of hatred toward the hatred (your relationship to
the attachment). You don't like the idea of being someone who hates.

*Step Four: Become intimate with the attachment and
your relationship to it.* Explore what resisting hating feels
like. Where is it in your body? What thoughts do you have
about it in your mind? What actions are you tempted to
take? Your intimacy with hatred and hating hatred lie at
the heart of the letting-go process. Your ability to make
peace with these experiences is what helps release you from
the hold they have on you.

Step Five: Notice what happens. Your attachments give
you the opportunity to develop patience and kindness toward them, and the grasping melts away. Then you are free
to choose the best response to the situation: what's really
best for you and also for others.

When you pay attention to the way hatred works (and the way hating hatred works), there's no struggle, there's no grasping, there's no clinging. If there's no struggle, there's no suffering. If there's no suffering, there's no problem. You are free to receive nourishment from hatred (or any other attachment) because the nourishment comes from your willingness to be fully in the present moment, no matter what it is.

BARRIERS TO LETTING GO

From birth, you are conditioned to relate things to yourself. You learn your name, where you live, who your parents are, and which toys are yours. These are important things to know in life because they help create the concept of who you think you are. You continuously add new concepts to who you imagine yourself to be: "I'm overweight," "I'm physically fit," "I'm a good cook," or "I'm a vegetarian," for example. Once the concepts become *me*, there's also the need to defend them, because that's who you think you are.

If you think you are a gourmet cook, you worry about how everything tastes. If you believe you're physically fit, you spend your time trying to stay that way. If you believe you're frightened of gaining weight, you obsess about what you put in your mouth.

But these descriptions of *me* are only concepts, and they survive only because you cling to them. The truth is they're not who you are because who you are is constantly changing. If you don't understand the temporary and fleeting nature of these descriptions, you struggle to make them permanent. This struggle to make these descriptions permanent is what makes letting go so difficult. You don't want to give up the idea of being someone who needs dessert after every meal, or give up the image of yourself as someone who makes the best apple crisp in town.

But the truth is that you don't really lose anything when you let go. Letting go of these concepts is like removing something that is imaginary. You can't *lose* these things because they weren't ever really yours. There is nothing that you own or possess for very long. Even your body does not belong to you, and it will die someday. So there's no point in identifying or claiming anything as your own, because nothing—not your body, not your idea of who you think you are, nor your next meal—is going to last.

Many patterns of behavior and self-image come from early childhood. Many others come from the various identities we have been given by others and those we've given to ourselves. But having an identity at one time doesn't mean it should last forever or even last at all. Eating everything on your plate may have been an identity you enjoyed as a child. But if that identity no longer serves you well and is the cause of suffering, learn how to let it go.

You can explore the feelings behind eating everything on your plate. These feelings may include the desire to please, the desire to be loved, or the desire to avoid punishment. Your willingness to become intimate with these feelings are the seeds of emotional nourishment. This intimacy gives you the chance to make peace with yourself by learning to open up to these feelings and enjoy the nourishment they offer. From that perspective, you can then make a decision about eating everything on your plate, depending on whether this serves you well or not. There's no need to focus on how rotten your parents were for forcing you to eat everything on your plate. That story just fuels the attachment. If someone shoots an arrow into your heart, it's useless to yell at the person. It's better to turn your attention to the wound and try to get the arrow out. That attention to the wound is at the center of letting go as well as the source of healing it.

STANLEY MILGRAM'S INSIGHTS

Stanley Milgram, the late social psychologist, conducted experiments on obedience to authority at Yale University in the 1960s. To everyone's surprise, participants obeyed the orders of the "authority" even though they were instructed to hurt another person with increasingly severe electric shocks. Most participants never questioned the authority. Instead, they obeyed the harmful commands.

Most of us have an inner authority telling us who we are (fat or thin, bad or good) and what to do (eat more or less, eat here or there). Like the participants in the Milgram experiments, we carry out the orders without questioning who's in charge. But that inner authority has no real power if you don't respond to it. It just fades away. You don't *have* to listen to that voice and do what it says, especially if it's not in your best interest. Instead of being driven by patterns and habits from the past, you can let go and be free to make wise choices in the present moment.

Milgram told a story that he imagined before he began the experiments on obedience to authority. Two men were walking down the street and were approached by a stranger. The stranger asked the two men to follow him, and they agreed. They were led into a building and taken to a small office. "Today is the day you're going to die," the stranger said. "You can either die by lethal injection or die by poison. Which do you prefer?" One man said, "I'll take the lethal injection." The other man simply walked out the door.

The first man blindly obeyed the authority of the stranger. The second man recognized it wasn't in his best interest to do so and walked away. This is exactly what you must learn to do in the letting-go process: Walk away from situations that are harmful or not in your best interest. This takes practice.

WHAT TO EXPECT

Letting go is not something you do once and say, "That's that." There is no instant way to let go. Even if you've examined your attachments to hatred or love many times, there are always new challenges to face. That's why letting go is considered a *practice* and why there's unlikely to be a book called *How to Let Go in Thirty Seconds*.

Habits related to strong emotions such as fear, loneliness, and anger are not easy to let go of. It's common to resist examining difficult patterns of behavior. Some habits are so powerful that when you let them go for a moment, you start to hold on even harder. For instance, you observe the tendency to be overly nice to someone who hasn't been very nice to you, and then see the desire to overeat shortly after that.

THERE'S SUFFERING AND FREEDOM FROM SUFFERING:
The Choice Is Yours

There's a tale about two monks who were great friends in a monastery and died within a few months of each other. One monk was reborn in a heavenly realm; the other was reborn as a worm. The monk in the heavenly realm looked for his friend but couldn't find him anywhere. Eventually, he found his friend in the animal realm, living as a worm in a pile of garbage.

The monk was determined to help his friend join him in the heavenly realm, so he went to visit him. But the worm told him to get lost. The monk tried to explain. "I am your friend. I can take you to an incredible place of beauty." The worm still didn't want to go. So the monk grabbed him and tried to pull him out of the garbage pile. The harder the monk tugged, the harder the worm clung to the garbage.

There's a little of that clinging worm in each of us. We get so accustomed to certain habits that even when we're given the opportunity to change, we don't take it. We become so comfortable with our habits that we want to stay as we are. We get comfortable with being angry or unhappy.

WENDY'S RESISTANCE

Wendy, a client in her late twenties, expected to go on a diet, lose weight, and live happily ever after. Wendy believed that losing weight would make her a kinder, gentler person, more graceful, lovely, and charming. But during the first several months that we worked together she said, "I never experienced so much hatred and anger in my life." She wondered why something she thought would be making her so happy was making her so miserable.

Raised to be a good girl, she saw strong emotions like anger as an enemy, something to be fought and conquered. Whenever Wendy felt anger or hatred, she'd whip out a doughnut or nibble on chips. Her self-image was one of a kind person who didn't hate anyone or anything. Even a *hint* of anger or unkindness was repressed.

As Wendy began losing weight, she became desperate for things to do. She looked for distractions, but intense feelings of anger and hatred overwhelmed her. She then began to wonder what was so terrible about being a good girl. She missed that role. After all, she was comfortable in it and it served her well for many years. To Wendy, the good-girl life seemed a lot more gentle than the angry life she was now living. She doubted her ability to change. But instead of buying into this self-doubt, *she noticed it.* She saw this feeling as an opportunity to explore her desire to return to a role she was more comfortable with. She noticed the tendency but didn't react to it. On some level, she knew that she couldn't go back to that role, anyway.

By staying with these feelings of doubt and resistance, the strong feelings subsided. She felt the feelings of doubt and resistance in her body and mind and realized how much grasping there was within her. They felt like a tight fist around her heart.

Wendy focused her attention on that feeling every time it came up. She practiced being patient and kind with it, rather than struggling against it. The more she became familiar with that feeling, the less compelled she was to distract herself by overeating. Wendy found that it was easier to feel anger and her resistance to it than it was to hold on to an outdated image of herself as a good girl and repress her feelings. She realized that by allowing feelings to come and go, they fade away on their own.

What you (or Wendy or Marilyn) do for yourself in the letting-go process—any gesture of kindness, any gesture of honesty and seeing clearly—will affect how you experience your world. In fact, it will transform how you experience the world. What you do for yourself you also do for others, and what you do for others, you do for yourself. When you're willing to go beneath your story line (of being a good girl or someone who fears rejection), you experience feelings that are experienced by all of us. In this way, when you practice letting go, you change yourself and your connection to the world you live in.

WAYS TO BE MINDFUL OF THE THIRD NOBLE TRUTH

1. Review the steps to letting go on pages 63–65 and practice letting go of:

- Complaining about your weight or your body
- Feeling bad when you don't get what you want

- The urge to eat when you're not hungry
- The desire to always be right
- Feeling not good enough

As you consciously let go of these feelings, notice:

- Where do you tend to get stuck?
- How can you be more kind and patient at this time?
- What would you want the person you love most in the world to do if he or she was in a similar situation?

2. Notice the food and eating habits that don't serve you well.

- What are they?
- What attachments are bonding you to them? Do you have to have dessert after every meal?
- What feelings are beneath that urge to have?
- Practice letting go one layer at a time. Examine your relationship to having to have? Is it grasping? Is it rejection? Is it fear?
- Feel these feelings within you, and then notice what happens. Does this change your relationship to having to have dessert after every meal?

3. Notice any resistance to letting go.

- Notice what habits you resist letting go of. For instance, is there resistance to giving up wanting to be right, or being angry at someone?
- What is motivating your resistance? Do you like the feeling that comes from being right? Do you believe that the person you're angry at deserves your anger?

• Notice how this resistance feels within you. Is it comfortable or not? Notice what happens to these feelings of resistance as you become more familiar with them.

4. Notice the nourishing qualities that you bring to letting go. Acknowledge qualities like kindness and patience as seeds of self-nourishment that are growing inside you. They are the antidotes to the feelings of emotional hunger that come from grasping and clinging.

CHAPTER 4

THE EIGHTFOLD PATH:

Guidelines for Ending Emotional Hunger

APPLYING THE FOURTH NOBLE TRUTH

◎

What, now, is the Noble Truth of the Path that leads to the extinction of suffering? It is the Noble Eightfold Path, the way that leads to the extinction of suffering.

—*The Buddha*

The Fourth Noble Truth is a further set of instructions about how to let go of suffering and experience emotional nourishment. It consists of eight sections, known as the Eightfold Path. The path explains the various and creative ways you can learn to let go and feel full. The Eightfold Path is called *the Middle Way* because it avoids the extremes of indulgence and deprivation that trigger emotional hunger within you.

It's helpful to think of each section of the path as a recipe for nourishing your heart. Unlike traditional recipes that focus on quantities of sugar or rice, these recipes use other nutrients that aren't usually found in cookbooks or in nutrition charts, such as gratitude, generosity, kindness, patience, and honesty. In fact, these recipes use *everything*, including sorrow and joy, and pain and pleasure to transform suffering/hunger into an enduring fullness.

Whether you are scrubbing vegetables, wiping crumbs off the dining room table, or eating a delicious piece of cake, you can use these recipes to nourish your heart and experience the kind of fullness that lasts.

Here are the aspects of the Eightfold Path, grouped in the three traditional sections:

WISDOM

1. Right Understanding
2. Right Aspiration

ETHICAL CONDUCT

3. Right Speech
4. Right Action
5. Right Way of Living

EMOTIONAL BALANCE

6. Right Effort
7. Right Mindfulness
8. Right Concentration

You may be wondering why the word *Right* appears before each aspect of the path. *Right* is the usual translation of the word *samma* in Pali (the language of the Buddha). The word indicates that certain behaviors can either lead to nourishment or suffering. For example, telling the truth (Right Speech) and feeling grateful (Right Action) help create peace within you and within the world, whereas telling lies and being selfish help create both inner and outer conflict. In short, the Eightfold Path points you in the right direction; it leads you toward fullness and away from hunger.

MINDFULNESS

Mindfulness is the basis of the Eightfold Path. As I mentioned earlier, mindfulness is known as the medicine that cures the disease of desire. When you pay attention to what's true in the moment (as you shop, cook, eat, or dance) that focused awareness slows you down long enough to examine your habits. If you *know* you're reaching for a chocolate chip cookie, that moment of mindfulness can break the automatic response to mindlessly put it in your mouth. This awareness helps cut through the compulsive habit of chasing desire after desire only to experience deeper and deeper levels of hunger. It offers you an opportunity to question what you want to do next, knowing that your decision can either create nourishment or suffering within you. Mindfully deciding to eat a cookie offers choices that aren't available to you when you are mindlessly operating on automatic pilot.

Being mindful focuses your attention on the things you

take for granted and don't bother to notice, like the stains on your teacup, the lose handle on the frying pan, or the delight of a bowl of hot soup on a cold day. These are the kinds of moments that often go unrecognized. Yet these are the ones that our lives are made up of, and which provide the *mindfulness* that comes from paying attention to the present without grasping.

Mindfulness helps you fall in love with the ordinary. Pounding the bottom of the ketchup bottle or wiping up a greasy stove may not be your idea of a dream come true, but unlike dreams, these experiences are real. They are what's true in our lives, meal after meal, day after day. When you are mindful of them, you discover that each time you do something, even if you've done the same thing a million times before, that moment is completely unique. It never happens twice. You can receive nourishment from each moment and become *mind full* of its presence. In other words, the present moment is an ongoing source of fullness, but you have to be aware of it to receive it.

To nourish your heart, you have to *practice* working with these recipes. They're not a one-time proposition; they're a lifetime commitment. There are always new things to discover and experiment with. Practicing Right Effort in one moment will be completely different in another moment, so there's always a new opportunity to apply your effort.

Since all the sections are related, when you practice one, you actually practice them all. For instance, practicing Right Action is also practicing Right Way of Living, which is also practicing Right Speech. They're contained within each other. No matter what recipe you practice, or what order you practice them in, you can always find suffering, the cause, and the way to end it.

Many great teachers have compared the Eightfold Path

to reading a cookbook, practicing the path to cooking food, and attaining peace to knowing the taste of food. If you simply read the recipes without putting them into practice, it's like knowing about peppers, onions, and garlic, but never knowing how they taste.

So please enjoy and feast on a lasting nourishment that can only be received by practicing them.

PART THREE

RECIPES FOR NOURISHING THE HEART

CHAPTER 5

RIGHT UNDERSTANDING:
Seeing the Truth in Everything

RECIPE #1

@

*And what is Right Understanding? Knowledge with regard to
suffering, knowledge with regard to the origin of suffering,
knowledge with regard to the way of practicing leading to the
end of suffering. This is called Right Understanding.*
—THE BUDDHA

Right Understanding is the first recipe and section of the
Eightfold Path. The nourishment you receive from
Right Understanding comes from realizing the truth of suffering, its cause, and how it ends in every moment of awareness. Any experience—wanting, never feeling satisfied, or
peeling a cucumber—can be used as an opportunity to understand and awaken to the Noble Truths. Here are some
examples:

1. When you find it impossible to change your eating habits, you can reflect on the nature of suffering and the fact that it includes both inevitable and optional suffering. You can remind yourself that how you react to an experience may be freely chosen, although the situation itself may not be.

2. When you want your salad served after the main course and not before it, you can reflect on the cause of suffering. You can acknowledge your attachment to wanting and see it separately from the desire itself.

3. When you really want a bowl of ice cream, even when you're not hungry, you can reflect on letting go. You can feel wanting within you and explore your relationship to those feelings.

When you're *mindful of your reaction*, you are acknowledging the First Noble Truth: that there is suffering. When you are *mindful of wanting things to be other than they are*, you are acknowledging the Second Noble Truth that explains the cause of suffering. When you are *mindful of letting go your attachment to desire* and your subjective response to it, you are acknowledging the Third Noble Truth: there is the end of suffering.

DARK FILTERS

Without Right Understanding, you see every thing through dark filters of desire. You can't see the truth of suffering, its cause, or how to end it, so you do things that perpetuate your emotional appetite by getting caught in an endless series of traps. The practice of Right Understanding helps remove the filters so you can see clearly again.

Without Right Understanding, you can't really appreciate the beauty of life. Although beauty is energizing and makes you feel connected, it's tinged with desire. There's grasping because you want to keep the good feeling going forever. Similarly, you can't appreciate suffering without Right Understanding. When you're suffering, you feel humbled and that there's nothing to lose. You're not caught up in supporting or defending a self-image. But if there's always suffering, you grasp by rejecting it and become demoralized by it.

With Right Understanding, you can see that beauty and suffering need each other. Appreciating the beauty of life energizes you, just as acknowledging the suffering in life softens you. This is a very important insight that comes from Right Understanding. When you see your attachment to beauty and suffering clearly, they reveal their frustrating nature and their inability to provide lasting happiness or sadness. That understanding helps you let go of them both. This is why the Buddha said, "Know the world. It's bedazzling like a king's royal carriage. Fools are entranced, but the wise are not deceived."

MARA: THE TEMPTER

Mara is the personification of things that get in the way of Right Understanding. Mara is the force that takes you out of the present by enticing you with something else, like a fantasy of the future (e.g., an urge for a bag of potato chips) or a longing from the past (e.g., the muffins you had last week). Mara comes in many forms: fear, anger, resistance, or as general unwillingness to look at what's true.

Mara's strong and persistent message tells you to forget about Right Understanding: hate that person or want that piece of cake or need a new flavor of olive oil. In whatever way Mara can, this force tries to get your attention away from what's going on right now. Without Right Understanding, it's easy to get lost in these distractions.

When Mara strikes, you feel like you're being attacked by a ruthless army. The expression *the armies of Mara* depicts this image. First you are attacked by *desire*. All you can think about is french fries. Then *attachment* sets in. You don't just want any old french fries, you want the long, thick ones with crinkles in them. Then *the thrill of the pursuit* sets in. You hope there's no traffic on the way to the supermarket so you can get them right away. Before you know it, *suffering in the form of emotional hunger and self-hatred* takes over. Won't you ever learn to keep boxes of french fries in the freezer? The armies keep attacking until you see them clearly.

Right Understanding is a matter of loving or hating Mara or trying to get rid of this force forever. Right Understanding offers the opportunity to awaken to Mara through mindfulness. You can transform the force of Mara into a source of nourishment by seeing Mara clearly.

There's no rational reason to be hard on yourself when you do get lost. As I discussed in the introduction, the armies of Mara visited the Buddha on the night of his enlightenment. He was besieged by Mara. But instead of getting caught up in these forces, he opened himself up to them and received the nourishment they offered. The Buddha was enlightenment by his ability to transform Mara through Right Understanding.

Actually, it can be a lot of fun (and I do mean *fun*) to share Mara experiences with friends. Telling Mara stories is a good way of releasing Mara's power over you. It's a way of acknowledging Mara as a habit rather than as a force that's concrete and resistant to change. You also get to see how ubiquitous Mara is. It's hard to find a time, place, or situation where Mara's presence isn't felt. Instead of feeling inadequate and defensive because you didn't have any Cajun food in New Orleans (or deep dish pizza in Chicago, or smoked salmon in Seattle), you can see the situation clearly and remind yourself, "There's Mara again."

WAYS TO BECOME MINDFUL OF RIGHT UNDERSTANDING

1. Use Right Understanding to see the Noble Truths in the following situations:

- When you feel obsessed with food
- When you're jealous of someone who isn't conflicted about food
- When you feel anxious about going to a party with a lot of tempting food
- When you love Italian or any other kind of food

2. Get to Know Mara, the tempter.

- Watch how Mara and the armies of Mara work. When is Mara most delightful? Most mischievous? Most devious? Most annoying?
- Find out what Mara is looking for. Safety? Security? Love? Acceptance?
- Notice what happens as you become more familiar with Mara.

CHAPTER 6

RIGHT ASPIRATION:

How Meaning Motivates

RECIPE #2

❂

*And what is Right Aspiration? Right Aspiration is being resolved
on renunciation, on freedom from ill will, and harmlessness. The
thinking, directed thinking, and focused awareness in one
developing the Noble Path whose mind is noble.
This is Right Aspiration.*
—THE BUDDHA

The second aspect of the Eightfold Path is Right Aspiration. It focuses on the importance of mental attitude. There are two sides of Right Aspiration. One is cultivating wholesome attitudes and behavior; the other is refraining from unwholesome attitudes and behavior. Right Aspiration also stresses the importance of placing eating in a meaningful context, so that it's not just another routine or unconscious activity in your day. When eating (or not eating) is connected to generosity and gratitude instead of how good you look or how thin you are, you receive a more lasting kind of nourishment.

ASPIRE, DON'T DESIRE

On the surface, Right Aspiration seems like a subtle form of desire: desiring positive attitudes and behaviors rather than negative ones. But there are subtle and important differences between desiring and aspiring.

Sankappa, a term in Pali, the language of the Buddha, means aspiration or a special kind of *desire in which there is clarity.* Sankappa recognizes that there's more to life than chasing one desire after another. It also acknowledges that there's a vast and sacred realm to tap into that supplies emotional nourishment instead of fuel for suffering.

Sankappa is expansive and inclusive. This kind of aspiration connects you to experiences and mysteries larger than your own self-interests and concerns. It invites you to be receptive to things and to wonder about the vastness of the universe. When you practice Right Aspiration, you feel in touch with the miraculous and the sacred. You're aware of things such as:

• The miracle of food: that it grows on trees, sprouts up from the ground, and gets to your table
• The miracle of the body: that you have a digestive, nutrient-absorbing, and elimination system that processes your food every day
• The miracle of nature: that an average ear of corn has 800 kernels arranged in sixteen rows

• The mystery of life: how a peach pit becomes a peach tree

• The contribution of each element to what we eat: earth, air, fire, and water

To have a more personal understanding of *sankappa*, take a quick look in the refrigerator and food cabinets in your house. You might be amazed to find cheese or mustard from France, basmati rice from India, stuffed grape leaves from Greece, maple syrup from Canada, strawberry jam from England, and olive oil from Italy. When you stop and reflect on this for a moment, it's really quite amazing. Just within the space of your kitchen, there's a whole range of cultures, traditions, weather conditions, and vast numbers of people involved. Appreciating all of this is *sankappa*. It helps bring your feeling about food to a higher level, out of the ordinary.

Tanha, another Pali term, is the opposite of *sankappa*. It means *a desire that comes out of confusion, of not seeing clearly*. The focus of *tanha* is self-centered. It encourages the pursuit of personal desires, even though taking more than your share and leaving others without may cause suffering. When you're *tanha*-focused (as many traditional diets encourage you to be), there's a lot of time spent evaluating:

• How fast you can get results

• How easy something (like losing weight) will be to accomplish

• How convenient something is

• If you will feel deprived

• If you will be bored

• If you can get more if you like it

ZEENA'S STORY

Zeena learned the important distinction between aspiration and desire in a dramatic way. While she was traveling in India, Zeena had to eat very simply. Fresh fruits and vegetables were rare, so was clean drinking water. Many people around her were starving and had to beg for food. Zeena then flew to New Zealand where she was treated to a welcome-to-the-country dinner by several friends. Within hours, she went from an extreme of deprivation to an extreme of abundance. The restaurant they ate in was elegant. Large portions of food were served—enough to feed several people by Indian standards. Zeena said, "I sat there in awe. Everything looked so great, clean, and wonderful. I was full of wonder and appreciation for what was in front of me." Then came the shock. Her hosts spent the evening criticizing everything they ate. The avocado wasn't ripe, the lamb was overcooked, the dessert cart didn't have enough choices, the wine was disappointing. She was shocked that her friends were blind to the privilege of their abundance and were so unappreciative of what they were eating.

Her friends were so focused on what was *wrong* with the meal that they missed how extraordinary it actually was. When you're wrapped up in how the experience impacts you, it's easy to miss the beauty of it. An important perspective is lost: eating is nothing to take for granted. The sharp contrast between what Zeena experienced eating in India and then in New Zealand provided a new sense of meaning for her, one that included appreciation and respect.

LINDA'S AWAKENING

Sometimes a life-threatening situation triggers a major shift in your attitude toward food and eating. Illness, disaster, and death can move us away from our ordinary, mundane concerns about how much we weigh and what we look like toward a more meaningful state of mind. This is more in tune with Right Aspiration.

While Linda was losing weight, she never stopped talking about it. She was totally absorbed in her diet, how much she had lost and how her clothes fit. Her main concern each day was whether or not she'd treat herself to a frozen yogurt. That narrow *tanha*-driven focus changed suddenly the day Linda came home and found her husband lying on the floor. He had suffered a major heart attack. Linda called an ambulance, and he was rushed to the hospital. For the next twenty-four hours, Linda didn't know if her husband would live or die. She sat by his bed in the intensive care unit, reflecting on their marriage. She remembered the first time they met, their first kiss, and when he proposed. Hours went by without a single thought about either her weight or her yogurt. She couldn't have cared less about them.

Ever since Linda's husband's heart attack and subsequent recovery, her focus has expanded. She's grateful and happy to be alive. Food is still important, but in a new way. She won't allow excess weight to take away the sense of joy she feels about the preciousness of life. Linda makes sure she looks up at the sky every day and feels the ground under her feet. She also complains less and spends more time with those most important to her. Linda's desire for a trim, healthy body has changed. She used to want to fit into an ideal image of beauty; now she has a profound appreciation of her body as it is and of being alive. Linda's husband's almost deadly heart attack opened up this realm of reality to her. It gave her life more depth and meaning and put her food problems in perspective.

THE TYRANNY OF CHOICE

One of the reasons it's so easy to be picky and at the same time oblivious to the abundance in our lives is our overabundance of choices. We thrash around in a sea of empty desires destined to change and then wonder why we're drowning.

Coffee
Types: regular, decaffeinated, house blend, special blend, water processed, light roast, dark roast, espresso, latte, mocha latte
Grind: coarse, medium coarse, medium fine, fine
Coffemaker: old-fashioned drip, percolator, plunger pot, flat-bottom filter, filter cone, espresso

Milk
Types: whole milk, 1 percent, 2 percent, no-fat, skim, buttermilk, cream, half-and-half, enriched milk, fresh acidophilus (regular and low-fat)

Bread
Types: white, whole wheat, organic whole wheat, pumpernickel, seven grain, nine grain, twelve grain, oatmeal, oatmeal and raisin, raisin, sourdough, semisourdough, rye (seeded or unseeded), dill, cheese, rosemary and tomato, pumpkin spice, almond, potato-rosemary, tomato garlic, oregano pesto, sun-dried tomato, sesame millet, banana nut

Airline Food
    Types: bland, diabetic, fruit plate, gluten-free, Hindu, high-protein, hypoglycemic, infant, kosher, lactose-free, low-calorie, low-carbohydrate, low-fat, Muslim, ovo-lacto-vegetarian, seafood plate, soft, sulfite-free, vegetarian, vegan vegetarian

Restaurants
    Types: fast-food, deli, take-out, cafeteria, family style, all-you-can-eat, drive-in, gourmet, nouvelle cuisine, ethnic, diner, steak house, coffee shop, pizza parlor, bar, ice cream parlor
    Styles: casual, formal, semiformal, charming, cozy, high-tech, stylish, elegant, charming

Diets
    Types: The I Love New York Diet, The Scarsdale Diet, Dr. Atkins Diet, The Beverly Hills Diet, The Eat to Win Diet, The Rice Diet, The Never Say Diet Diet, The Cambridge Diet, The Long Weekend Diet, The Runner's Diet, The Popcorn Diet, The Steak and Salad Diet, The Choose to Lose Diet, The Carbohydrate Addict's Diet, The Vacation Diet, The Blender Diet, Beyond Dieting, The One-Day Diet

LOOK AT WHAT'S GOOD

One evening when Rachel was visiting some friends, she casually said, "I never worry about my weight." This comment amazed the other dinner guests. "How do you manage that?" was what everyone wanted to know.

"It's easy. I think about food as sacred, not as a way to make myself feel better," Rachel responded. "I was in a Nazi concentration camp during World War II. I was a very young child, separated from my parents, brothers, and sister, who died there. I was the only one in my family of nine to survive. People in the camp were starving to death all around me; no one ever got enough to eat, including me. Even so, I often gave away my food and therefore ate even less than everyone else. My parents were religious and ate only kosher food, so when I was in the camp, I kept kosher. It wasn't a problem for me to turn down food, even when I was hungry, which was pretty much all the time. Trying to keep kosher in this horrendous situation helped preserve my family's memory in my heart; it gave me a strength I didn't even know I had."

Rachel's comments dramatically affected the other dinner guests. If Rachel could turn down food in the face of starvation, why was it so hard for them to turn down second helpings or an afternoon snack?

RESTRAINT AND FREEDOM

There's a place in all of us that knows that anything worthwhile often requires restraint and a certain amount of sacrifice. It's no coincidence that so many religious practices require discipline around food. There's satisfaction in knowing that what you eat (or don't eat) actually means something more than how it is going to affect a number on the scale or how your clothes fit. Restraint comes more naturally when you are connected to more than just what food tastes like and how much it is or isn't going to satisfy you.

Fasting, for instance, is symbolic of purification and strengthening one's religious commitment. During Ramadan, Muslims fast as a way to engender empathy for those hungry for food as well as for those hungry for spiritual connection. To symbolize self-purification of the heart, they refrain from frivolous activities such as gossip and exaggeration. These disciplines help redirect attention and energy toward the sacred instead of the profane.

KARIMA'S PERSPECTIVE

Karima feels that fasting for Ramadan gives her a sense of purification. She enjoys the sense of vulnerability. "I'm not invincible," she admits. "I need food. I especially like the evening or day after a fast. Then when I eat I really appreciate what food tastes like. It's so good. I don't feel that sense of appreciation when I can eat whatever I want, whenever I want it. Eating loses its meaning if there are no fasting days. I don't have the same motivation to give up food when I'm trying to lose weight. Fasting for religious purity makes sense; eating less to reduce my body weight makes sense, too. It just doesn't have the same meaning."

RESTRAINT CAN FEEL GOOD

Anne has always taken Lent (the forty days before Easter) very seriously. Practicing Catholics make sacrifices to remind themselves of the sacrifices that Christ made on their behalf. Anne makes good use of this time and spends time reflecting on what to give up. She wants to make a real sacrifice; she enjoys making the deep commitment. "Everyone in the community takes their sacrifice seriously," Anne explains. "People look down on you if you give up something you rarely eat anyway, like caviar or porcini mushrooms. It's better to give up something you eat all the time, like cookies or butter. That's really making a sacrifice and connecting to the spirit of the holiday. Otherwise, giving up something is meaningless."

During Lent, Anne never has the difficulties she has when she tries to lose weight. "Restraint during Lent makes me feel good about myself," she says. "Restraint when I'm trying to lose weight makes me feel terrible. I walk around feeling like a deprived two-year-old. I want what I want, and I want it now!"

DIETARY LAWS

Religious Jews and Muslims follow strict dietary laws that spell out what and when certain foods can and cannot be eaten. In other words, they must be mindful of what they eat. Muslims and Jews don't eat pork; Jews avoid combining milk and meat. They must ask themselves before they eat: Is this kosher? If the answer is no, they don't eat it. These dietary laws help expand their spiritual commitment into their daily lives. Since eating happens several times a day, moments of mindfulness are built into the daily lives of those who follow these laws. The motivation behind this commitment to discipline is very different from the one that drives us to want to look good in a bathing suit or to conform to an ideal image of beauty. Consequently, there's a different relationship to restraint.

WHEN FOOD HAS MEANING

Shana follows Jewish dietary laws because she believes they are commanded by God. She doesn't see them as complicated or inconvenient; to her they're holy and meaningful. This fills more than just her physical appetite.

Yet when Shana decides to cut back on certain foods because she wants to lose weight, she's rarely successful. "I never have the willpower to stay on a diet," she says. "Not eating something because I'm trying to lose weight involves my vanity and is very limited in scope. On the other hand, breaking a fast or one of the dietary laws would have cosmic consequences. These laws are part of the bond I have with God, and breaking any one of them would affect our relationship in a serious way. I wouldn't even think of doing that. What I eat or don't eat goes beyond just me. It's my relationship to everything I believe in."

Marvin also adheres to the Jewish dietary laws. He says that every time he eats, he naturally questions, "What am I eating? Does this fit into a larger framework that connects me with all of life?" He continues, "The main reason I diet is to be more attractive. It's not a holy goal. I feel conflicted by it. It doesn't connect me to the deepest truth of my being. I'm annoyed at myself that it even matters and that there's a large part of me that wants to be more attractive. This desire is not connected to a transcendent purpose, and so it brings up a lot of ambivalence within me."

It takes more than a desire to make changes in your behavior. It also takes putting these changes into a meaningful context. If the context is not meaningful enough, turning down food is difficult. On the other hand, when refusing food has meaning, it seems easier, as it has been for Rachel, Karima, Anne, Shana, and Marvin. Giving up foods helped them feel full, not deprived. What they ate (or didn't eat) had significance. It offered them a form of nourishment that physical food could not provide. They were motivated by a larger aspiration, one that was higher than the desire to feel full or please themselves.

On the other hand, when the purpose of restraint relates only to weight loss, you're motivated by *tanha,* a confused desire that has no relationship to changing or improving your life in a larger context. The control of food for your own sake is ultimately less satisfying and a less powerful motive than the control of food that links you to sources of meaning in life. These sources of meaning clearly provide a critical source of nourishment. The need to find meaning is important to everyone's life, not just to those involved in food and eating issues. Giving meaning can help raise the most mundane activity, like scraping the grease off a frying pan, to a situation that feels precious and sacred.

THE IMPORTANCE OF FLEXIBILITY

Right Aspiration encourages you to find the special meaning that will help motivate you to follow a set of guidelines, eating or otherwise. The specific guidelines themselves are much less important than the nature of the force behind them. Sometimes rules might conflict with aspirations. That's when personal judgment on how to best handle the situation is essential. For instance, monks aspire to living a kind, moral, and helpful life. But one of the rules some monks also live by is not handling food. The purpose of this rule is to reinforce the interdependence between monks and their lay supporters. Monks depend on the community for their physical nourishment, just as the community depends on monks for their emotional nourishment. A monk once told me about a situation in which his larger aspiration to help others conflicted with the rule of conduct regarding not handling food.

The monk was taken to a soup kitchen in Oakland, California, because he wanted to learn more about the problem of hunger and homelessness in the United States. This particular soup kitchen serves breakfast to about sixty homeless men a day. The monk was so inspired by the generosity of the volunteers and the needs of the recipients that he started scrambling eggs, loading the toasters, and serving the meal. Another monk looked on critically, believing his friend was breaking an important rule. With a pan full of scrambled eggs in his hand, the cooking monk said, "It's far more appropriate to help others in this situation than it is to obey a rule that's not appropriate to it."

Right Aspiration isn't about blind obedience to an arbitrary sets of rules, like following a grapefruit low-protein diet. It's about giving meaning to your behavior, no matter what the rules are. There's no point in following rules if they're going to hurt you or someone else. It may be very appropriate to turn down a piece of cake because you don't eat dessert. In another situation, when a friend has gone to great lengths to bake you a cake for your birthday, the same response may be unwise. This is something you must work out for yourself. Following guidelines and exercising restraint are important, but so is flexibility.

FOOD AS SYMBOLS

Another way to bring a deeper meaning to what you eat is to learn more about what certain foods symbolize. When you are mindful of them, your relationship to this food often changes. You feel differently about the food because you have a connection to what it represents. The Eucharist, the blood and body of Christ, for example, is symbolized by the wine and the wafer, which gives the experience of receiving them a more tangible quality. At the beginning of the Jewish New Year, it's customary to dip apple slices in honey to symbolize the wish for a sweet year. Another Jewish food custom is to bring round or oval-shaped food, like eggs and lentils, to people in mourning. This shape symbolizes the circular nature of life, which includes the cycles of birth and death. Eating these foods reminds mourners of this truth, which can easily get lost in the grip of grief.

COMFORT FOODS

Food doesn't have to take on religious meaning in order to have significance. It may be useful for you to consider what foods offer you comfort or what foods have special meaning to you. My friend Elizabeth speaks proudly about her family's tradition of cocoa and cinnamon toast at bedtime. This combination of food has been in her family for three generations, and she hopes the tradition will be passed on for

many more. For Marina, comfort food is a grilled cheese
sandwich and a cup of tea. "No matter what I'm feeling,
eating a grilled cheese sandwich always makes me feel better." The type of food really isn't as important as the meaning ascribed to it, such as a connection to family identity
and the ability to comfort oneself.

DEDICATION OF MERIT

Another way to give eating and the difficulties you have
with food more meaning is by dedicating merit. This is the
practice of offering any benefit that comes from your commitment to healthful eating to specific people or groups of
people. In Buddhism, dedication of merit is a form of generosity. You share any benefits that may come from your
actions with others instead of holding on to them for yourself. If you know your actions might help someone in some
way, you may be more motivated to do the best you can.
Your actions have consequences, whether you are aware of
them or not. My friend who is a cancer survivor dedicates
any merit she may receive from healthful eating to her husband and daughter. "What I put in my body is my future,
and my future affects my family. It's easy for me to eat well
because what I eat includes the people I love the most."

There are many creative ways to dedicate merit that can
bring more meaning to your relationship to food. Pregnant
women and their partners can dedicate merit that comes
from healthful eating to their unborn child. Heart attack
survivors can dedicate merit that comes from regular exercise to their grandchildren. You can dedicate merit that
comes from eating more fresh fruit and vegetables to the

farmers at the outdoor market, the soil, sun and rain, to all that helped nourish you. Here are some other examples:

MERIT FROM:	CAN BE DEDICATED TO:
Donating food or working in a soup kitchen	Hungry people everywhere
Being mindful of your Hungry Ghost	The Hungry Ghost in everyone
Cutting back on red meat	Heart disease and cancer patients
Doing weight-bearing exercise	Women with weak bones
Making a pot of soup for an elderly friend	Older people who live and eat alone
Losing or maintaining weight	Those suffering from eating problems

GRATITUDE

Cultivating gratitude is also helpful in giving food more meaning. Gratitude helps keep your heart open. You are filled with appreciation for what you have instead of being preoccupied with what you don't have or how deprived you feel. Oscar Wilde said, "After a good meal, one can forgive anybody, even one's relatives."

The opportunity to enjoy food with friends and family is precious. So is the opportunity to celebrate happy occasions like birthdays, anniversaries, and holidays. To be in the presence of love and abundance is nothing to take for granted. So many things have to happen in order to create them. Don't waste this valuable time to complain or criticize. Look for what's good, and you'll find a lot to be grateful for.

A food critic once told me that she finds it annoying when people don't acknowledge how lucky they are to have so much abundance and choice in their lives. "I don't care if someone has been a vegan for twenty years or how tired they are of nouvelle cuisine," she says. "When I'm eating with them, I wish they'd just be quiet, eat what is served, and be grateful for it."

MAGIC CARROTS

Elaine practices mindful eating. She recalls that when she ate everything in sight, she never really *appreciated* any of it. "I took it all for granted," she said. "As I began to change my eating habits and eat more healthfully, I developed a deep appreciation for carrots: their intense orange color, their sweetness, and their versatility. While shopping one day, it occurred to me that no matter how long I lived, it wouldn't be long enough to try all the ways to use and prepare carrots. I felt tears coming when I realized this was true for every single fruit and vegetable in the store. My tears were not just tears of gratitude. They were tears of grief for all the years I didn't appreciate how lucky I was."

FOOD BLESSINGS AS
EXPRESSIONS OF GRATITUDE

You can initiate occasions that invoke a sense of gratitude: saying grace or a blessing before and/or after a meal, for example. A few simple words of thanks, privately or with those present, are all it takes. Even if you're not especially religious (or you're not religious at all), you may find that a brief pause before eating is good. It helps make a connection to what you're about to eat and to the amazing chain of events that led to this meal. Some people hold hands, recite a special blessing, or sit in silence for a few minutes. The exact form of gratitude doesn't really matter. It's your commitment to expressing gratitude that gives eating more meaning. Here are some ways others have found to express gratitude. Perhaps they will be of inspiration to you.

Thich Nhat Hanh

Thich Nhat Hanh, a Vietnamese monk and head of the Plum Village community in France, recites this five-part blessing throughout a meal:

1. **As food is served:**
I see clearly the presence of the entire universe supporting my existence.
2. **While looking at a full plate of food:**
All living beings are struggling for life. May they all have enough food to eat today.
3. **Just before eating:**
The plate is filled with food. I am aware that each morsel is the fruit of much hard work by those who produced it.
4. **While taking the first four mouthfuls of food:**
With the first taste, I promise to practice loving-kindness.
With the second, I promise to relieve the suffering of others.
With the third, I promise to see others' joy as my own.

With the fourth, I promise to learn the way of nonattachment and equanimity.

5. **Upon finishing the meal:**

My plate is empty. My hunger is satisfied. I vow to live for the benefit of all beings.

Saint Francis

A well-known blessing comes from Saint Francis of Assisi, who lived in the early thirteenth century. He took all of his belongings, including what he was wearing, and gave them to the poor. He walked naked around the streets of Assisi until people brought him things to wear. Eventually, he established the order of Franciscans, which still exists today. This prayer begins with Lord, but you can substitute any name such as Creator, Life, World, or Mother Earth. This is Saint Francis's prayer:

Lord, make me an instrument of your peace.
Where there is hatred, let me sow love;
where there is injury, pardon;
where there is doubt, faith;
where there is darkness, light;
and where there is sadness, joy.

O Divine One, grant that I may not so much seek to be consoled as
*   to console;*
to be understood as to understand;
to be loved as to love,
For it is in giving that we receive,
it is in pardoning that we are pardoned,
and it is in dying that we are born to eternal life.

A Zen Grace

Innumerable labors brought us this food,
May we know how it comes to us.
Receiving this offering,
Let us consider whether our virtue and
Practice deserve it.
Desiring the natural order of mind,
Let us be free from greed, hate, and delusion.
We eat to support life and to practice
The way of the Buddha.

This food is for the three treasures,
For our teachers, family, and all people,
And for all beings in the six worlds.
The first portion is for the precepts,
The second is for the practice of concentration.
The third is to save all beings.
Thus we eat this food and awaken with everyone.

A Protestant Grace

For what we are about to receive, may the Lord make us truly
thankful.

A Jewish Grace

*Blessed is the Lord, Creator of the universe, who
sustains the entire world with goodness, kindness, and mercy.*

Our ruler gives food to all creatures, with mercy everlasting.

*Through abundant goodness we have never yet been in want;
may we never be in want of substance for the sake of the Creator's
name.*

*The Lord sustains all, does good to all, and provides food for all.
Blessed is the Creator, who provides food for all.*

A Common Grace

The following grace is used in many Western cultures. In
a few short lines it conveys the importance of nourishing
both the emotional and physical aspects of hunger.

> *Bless this food we are about to receive.*
> *Give bread to those who hunger;*
> *and hunger for justice to us who have bread.*

WAYS TO BECOME MINDFUL OF RIGHT ASPIRATION

1. What food symbols and traditions are important to you? How can you integrate them in how you cook, shop, and eat so that you feel more connected to and inspired by these experiences?

2. Learn more about the culture, history, and origins of food and food traditions.

- What is halva and where does it come from?
- Do watermelons really come in yellow and white as well as pink and seedless?
- Where and when was broccoli first grown?
- What food customs do religious Greeks or Norwegians follow?
- What is the history of rhubarb?

3. Make a commitment to saying grace and/or dedicating merit at every meal, for one month. Notice what impact this practice has on your relationship toward food and its meaning in your life.

4. Experiment. Create your own grace before and/or after meals, depending on what you find most inspiring and meaningful. For a useful resource, refer to *One Hundred Graces*, selected by Marcia and Jack Kelly (Bell Tower Books, 1992).

CHAPTER 7

RIGHT SPEECH:
Filling Up by Speaking Right

RECIPE #3

◎

And what is Right Speech? Abstaining from lying, from divisive speech, from abusive speech, and idle chatter. Speaking to the truth, holding to the truth, and no deceiver of the world. This is called Right Speech.
—THE BUDDHA

Right Speech, the third aspect of the Eightfold Path and the third recipe for nourishing your heart, concerns speaking only what is true and useful. This kind of speech offers a feeling of inner fullness because it shows respect for yourself and others. Right Speech also means refraining from lying, slander, using harsh or critical words, and gossip. This kind of speech creates suffering and emotional hunger because it depletes your self-respect and the respect that others have for you.

Practicing Right Speech can be challenging. Have you ever:

- Made fun of someone's cooking?
- Been rude to a food server or grocery clerk?
- Told anyone that he or she looks better (or worse) than you really think?
- Described yourself or anyone else as a slob, or as big as a house?
- Described a particular food or dish as disgusting, horrible, sickening, or pathetic?
- Exaggerated how good or bad something tasted?
- Minimized the amount of an ingredient you used (e.g., butter, oil, cream)?
- Taken credit for something you didn't cook yourself?

If you have, you're not alone. That's why Right Speech is included among these recipes. It acknowledges the power of speech to create suffering or nourishment, depending on how it's used. Zen master Robert Aitken captures the essence of Right Speech when he says, "Self-deception, deception of others, cheating, gossip, and carelessness with language are all disloyal to the peace in our heart of hearts."

Right Speech flows naturally from Right Understanding and Right Aspiration. If you deeply understand the nature of suffering and how it can be transformed through gratitude and transcending personal desires, you naturally appreciate the importance of Right Speech. Within the Eightfold Path, it is viewed as a form of ethical conduct. Right Speech is considered one of the basic rules of decent human conduct, whereas sloppy speech is considered disruptive to the kind of conduct that creates peace and harmony within ourselves and within the world.

THE POWER OF WORDS

Speech is extremely powerful. It can be helpful or destructive, full of wisdom or venom. It can create a feeling of emotional destitution or a feeling of deep satisfaction. Consider the difference between calling someone sweetheart or darling and calling that person a jerk or beast, or imagine the difference between describing pudding as velvety smooth or as tasteless as flour and water. With a few words you can glorify or condemn anything. All of these words *feed back* to you and either add or deplete your nourishment supply.

There's a story about a meditation master who was asked to heal a sick child by saying some short prayers. A skeptic expressed doubt about the healing power of words. The master replied, "What do you know? You're an ignorant fool." The skeptic became enraged and shook with anger. Before he could reply, the master said, "If a few words can upset you so, why can't a few other words heal this sick child?"

Speech has consequences, so it's important to take responsibility for what you say. Otherwise, you run the risk of creating more and more suffering for yourself and for others. If you say something mean or untrue, you feel guilty and badly about yourself. These bad feelings multiply when other people's feelings get hurt by your words. Rumors may spread, and even more people may suffer. This is why the essential practice of Right Speech is to encourage everyone to please use words with the greatest care.

CARRIE'S STORY

Carrie has struggled with her weight all her life. She easily recalls the pain and humiliation she endured as an overweight child. On the playground and in the classroom, she was called fatso, tub of lard, and Dumbo. These labels were devastating to her. Carrie was unable to protect herself from the cruel remarks because she believed them. The abusive language spoken by others became the part of the foundation of her negative self-image.

It took Carrie many tears and lots of years to work out the emotional pain she held in her body and mind as a result of this kind of speech. Carrie's sensitivity to the damage of harsh speech helped her to become more mindful of her own use of speech. Paying careful attention to how she spoke to herself and to others had a profound impact on her. She saw all the ways she condemned herself, was critical of others, and the suffering these habits generated.

One of the most important lessons Carrie learned was to pay attention to what was driving her to speak critically. For instance, she realized that she criticized others when she was feeling insecure within herself. Instead of acting out her insecurity and spreading her own suffering, she now addresses that feeling inside of herself. She doesn't have to project her weaknesses on anyone else; she can see the strengths of others without feeling diminished within herself. When she responds to her own feelings of insecurity, she feels more nourished and more motivated to use Right Speech.

The motivation that lies behind speech is the source of whether your words create hunger or nourishment within yourself and others. When you're mindful of your motivation as Carrie was, you realize that a lot of speech is motivated by internal feelings of insecurity. If you want to look good, or build up your self-image to impress a colleague, you may exaggerate your accomplishments or experiences. There's no opportunity for nourishment through speech if you ignore the suffering that is motivating it. You'll continue to suffer and cause suffering to others.

On the other hand, acknowledging and responding to your own insecurity are forms of generosity to yourself that, in turn, promote generous speech from others. The more Carrie became intimate with her own insecurity, the more natural it was for her to speak in a supportive and helpful way to herself and to others.

She now enjoys the good feelings that come from complimenting and being supportive to friends because she's not as threatened by their accomplishments as she was when she was unaware of her own insecurities. Carrie also receives nourishment from being open and sincere with friends when they feel bad about themselves or a particular situation. Her ability to express genuine empathy to her friends and say things like, "I know how you must feel," helps them feel less alienated and at the same time helps Carrie feel more connected. She realizes that the ability to discover and become familiar with her own wounds is the grateful feeling nourished by the integrity that comes from this investigation.

FOUR RED FLAGS:
Lying, Slander, Critical Speech, and Gossip

Lying

Lying means intentionally misleading someone. Some lies can be quite bold, like pretending to find an insect in your food because you want to get a free meal. A lot of other lies are less calculating, but they're harmful and depleting, nonetheless.

A flight attendant learned that misleading someone can easily trigger a tremendous amount of suffering, even though at the time it seemed like no big deal. A passenger asked the flight attendant if there were any pine nuts in what was being served for dinner. She said, "I'll check," but she never did. When the passenger asked again, she lied. "There aren't any pine nuts in your food," she said. In fact, there were some nuts ground into the rice. The passenger, who was highly allergic to pine nuts, ate the rice and developed a severe, life-threatening reaction. The pilot had to make an emergency landing so the passenger could receive immediate medical attention. This incident caused a tremendous amount of suffering in the flight attendant who felt terribly guilty, to the passenger who got terribly sick, and to her family and the other passengers and crew members who got worried and scared.

Self-deception is another form of lying and a cause of tremendous suffering. You lie to yourself in order to avoid facing the truth. You might say things like, "I'll start exercising tomorrow," or "I'll stop nibbling between meals," even though you know on some level that these are hollow statements. Self-deceptions perpetuate suffering in many ways. They may sound genuine when, in fact, they are not. The gap between the self-deception and the truth triggers deep feelings of emptiness and hunger. Without self-understanding of what is generating the need to be self-deceptive, this habit of lying to yourself goes on and on and the possibility of self-nourishment becomes less and less.

Sometimes lying involves the *absence* of words. For instance, you receive a compliment on a dish that you didn't make and accept the credit for it anyway. Or you allow others to think that you made something when, in fact, you bought it. A client recalls how she brought a cake to a baby shower about forty miles from where she lives. Everyone raved about it. She accepted the compliment and never revealed it was a store-bought cake. Then another guest from the same town arrived late. Upon seeing the cake, she announced: "That bakery makes the best chocolate cake. We had the same delicious one last night." My client was embarrassed and felt depleted as a result of being caught in a lie, but the point that lies create a lot of suffering became crystal clear to her.

Slander

Slander creates mistrust by *intentionally* setting out to make someone look bad. For example, if you're upset that someone you don't like gets a prestigious job and then you tell the employer that this person isn't trustworthy, that's slander. You are intentionally saying something harmful to diminish someone in the eyes of another person.

Critical Speech

Critical speech also involves intention. Instead of the intention to create mistrust between people, the intention is to inflict harm through words. Critical speech runs from out-and-out cruel remarks such as, "You make me sick," to more subtle forms like, "Put on a few pounds lately?"

Both slander and critical speech have the potential to create enormous amounts of suffering. Although the wounds from a verbal attack are invisible, the suffering they cause can be greater than a physical attack. Someone's integrity or self-esteem isn't necessarily depleted by a punch or a slap, but mean or spiteful words often have the power to generate that kind of harm.

Slander and critical speech also erode your self-respect and the respect other people have for you. It's impossible to feel good about yourself when you intentionally hurt someone else. It's a cheap thrill with an expensive price tag. You are faced with the guilt and remorse that comes from speaking this way. Why should anyone trust you if you speak harshly to them or about someone else? Even if the person you're talking about isn't there or isn't listening, your insults can easily get back to the person you're putting down.

Evelyn's Chopped Liver

Evelyn stopped speaking to her sister Shirley because of a critical remark Shirley casually made at a family gathering. Shirley commented that Evelyn's chopped liver, an established family treasure, was "a little on the dry side this time." This infuriated Evelyn who, in turn, lashed back at Shirley by saying, "Who are you to criticize my chopped liver? All you ever make is a crummy Jell-O mold with fake whipped cream and canned fruit." Their critical remarks to each other were a source of great pain for over a year.

The suffering that follows as a result of critical speech can last a long time, even within a long-term marriage. In the case of Betty and Ted, it's lasted almost half a century. Even though the couple knows that certain topics trigger critical speech and then feelings of emptiness and hunger, they can't seem to stay away from them. The pattern is this: Betty and Ted reminisce about pivotal experiences that involved food: the ice cream soda they shared on their first date, the twelve-inch grilled hot dog they enjoyed at Coney Island, the lemon ice they ate every night on their first trip to Italy. It's only a matter of time until Ted brings up Betty's mother's cooking.

"I'll never forget the first meal I had at your house," he reminds his wife of forty-six years. "Your mother was the world's worst cook. You're lucky I still wanted to marry you."

His wife is not and has never been amused.

"What about *your* mother?" his wife replies as if they'd never had this conversation before. "She always put down my cooking and made nasty comments like, 'This jam isn't bad. Did it come in a jar?' Wherever I shopped, another place was *always* better."

Even though the conversation is predictable, Betty still feels hurt when her husband uses critical speech related to her mother's cooking. In fact, she told him, "The best present you could give me is never mentioning my mother's cooking again." Betty was offering Ted the chance to be generous. She was telling him that the absence of critical speech is a great gift.

Ellen's Feedback

Ellen realized that the *presence of generous speech* is also a great gift. Ellen put herself through college and architecture school working part time as a waitress. Over the years, she had her share of insults and abuse from demanding customers: "Come on, honey, you've got a hungry man on your hands here. Hurry up with my food." Others were not as crude but no less insulting: "Do you have lead at the bottom of your shoes?"

Now that Ellen's waitress days are over and she has made it as an architect, she makes it a practice to compliment food servers. She likes to acknowledge their hard work and express her appreciation for it. This small gesture of practicing generous speech feeds back a tremendous amount of nourishment. "Everyone likes to receive a compliment, especially food servers. Most of the time all they ever hear are complaints. One waitress followed me out the door to return the tip I left on the table. She said that my acknowledgment of her hard work was the real tip and the biggest one she had ever received."

Ellen's friends who see and hear the results of these compliments have picked up the habit of generous speech. They've been inspired to make the extra effort to be kind to food servers and to compliment them when the service is efficient and pleasant. Like Ellen, her friends feast on positive responses they get back in return. Both women hope that this practice will continue to spread and create nourishment for everyone involved.

Gossip

Gossip is the fourth red flag. Gossip is frivolous, mean-spirited talk, like discussing how bad the food was at a birthday party or how much weight someone has gained. Gossip hurts people. Sharing private information that's meant to stay private demeans the person who gossips and betrays the person he or she is talking about.

Emily's Speech Lesson
A colleague of Emily's told her in confidence that she was going to a residential weight reduction clinic for two weeks. The colleague made it very clear to Emily that she didn't want to deal with any pressure or expectations from the people at work, so Emily was to tell no one about where she was going. But one day while Emily was exchanging office gossip with a few other people, she told them about her colleague's visit to the weight reduction clinic. Upon her return to work, the colleague was bombarded with the questions she had hoped to avoid: "How much weight did you lose?" "Did you meet anybody famous?" "How was the food?"

Emily tried apologizing to her colleague, but the woman was too upset to even listen. She avoided Emily for a few weeks, and finally she told Emily how angry and betrayed she felt. The most painful part for Emily was hearing her colleague say, "I forgive you, but I'll never trust you with a secret ever again."

Like many lessons in life, the hardest ones have the most impact and offer the biggest opportunities for change. Emily has a new and more respectful relationship to the information people tell her in confidence. Instead of sharing idle gossip, Emily feasts on the good feelings she gets from protecting the trust others have put in her and that she now puts in herself.

NOT SWALLOWING LIES

Another important aspect of Right Speech is refusing to go along with lies that you know are untrue. If someone lies about serving low-fat ice cream when you know it is really regular (high-fat) ice cream, you speak up and don't go along with the lie.

Refusing to swallow lies is a difficult practice. How do you respond wisely, knowing that lies are part of our culture? The most important step to take is for each person to make a commitment to honest speech.

Food Companies' Lies

It's difficult to know how to respond when you are constantly bombarded with advertising lies, deceptions, and exaggerations. For instance, that the box of cereal you've been paying more for actually contains less cereal, or the fruit juice you're giving the children actually contains no fruit at all (it's fruit-flavored juice). These kinds of experiences cheapen human relationships and breed dishonesty and mistrust.

You can practice Right Speech by writing to the company executives and telling them that you don't appreciate these kinds of techniques that breed suspicion and mistrust. You can also learn to become your own authority so you rely less on advertisements and more on your own food and nutrition knowledge. For instance, terms like multigrain, sprouted wheat mean little or nothing on bread labels. If you want whole-grain bread that's high in fiber, the label must list whole wheat or another whole grain as the first ingredient; otherwise, it's mostly white flour. Similarly, advertising claims about weight loss require a lot of scrutiny. Just because someone lost fifty pounds in six weeks doesn't improve your odds. You don't know whether the person kept the weight off over the long haul or if the person gained it all back and more.

Make a commitment to gathering information from *unbiased publications* that don't accept advertisements from food companies, or any type of advertisements at all. Two of my favorite resources are:

1. *Tufts University Health & Nutrition Letter* (published monthly). Subscriptions are $24 per year. Write to: Box 57857, Boulder, CO 80322-7857.

2. *University of California at Berkeley Wellness Letter* (published monthly). Subscriptions are $28 per year. Write to: Box 420148, Palm Coast, FL 32142.

WAYS TO BECOME MINDFUL OF RIGHT SPEECH

1. Be meticulous in your speech. Say only what is true and useful. This can be a profound investigation. Notice

the impact it has on how you feel about yourself when you make the effort to choose your words wisely.

2. Make a commitment to refrain from talking about food-related topics for a week, and notice the impact this has on you. Notice whether it's easy or challenging, or if it's a relief or a burden.

3. Examine what motivates your desire to lie, slander, be critical, or gossip. Fear? The desire to be liked? The desire for power? Focus on the source of the suffering that lies behind this kind of speech, and notice what effect this has on the way you speak.

4. Practice generous speech. Make an effort to compliment and express your gratitude to those people you see working hard and who make a difference in your life and the lives of the people you care about.

5. Enjoy speech. Conversation can be a source of nourishment. Practicing Right Speech can help make this even more satisfying. Be generous, offer compliments, give accurate feedback, listen carefully.

CHAPTER 8

RIGHT ACTION:
Helping Others
as You Help
Yourself

RECIPE #4

◎

*And what is Right Action? The abstaining, abstinence,
avoidance, of the three forms of bodily misconduct (killing,
stealing, misconduct in relationships) in one developing the noble
path whose mind is noble, whose mind is without effluents, who is
fully possessed on the noble path. This is Right Action.*
—THE BUDDHA

Right Action, the fourth aspect of the Eightfold Path,
focuses on developing skillful behavior that grows out
of wisdom. This wisdom helps transform how you think.
For instance, you see the huge difference between inevitable
and optional suffering; you recognize the relationship between grasping and suffering. In turn, these insights transform your actions, just as your actions transform the way
you think.

The process and practice of changing your relationship to food falls under the umbrella of Right Action. Every time you pay attention to the present, you practice Right Action. There's no action more skillful than seeing things *exactly as they are* instead of how you might prefer them to be. It's a radical step away from always seeing through the dark filters of desire. But Right Action goes beyond this. It also involves your relationship to yourself, to your community, and to the environment we all share. Here are some examples of how to practice Right Action related to food and eating:

- Volunteer in a soup kitchen or food giveaway program.
- Support local farmers by buying what they grow.
- Learn more about nutrition so you rely less on advertising.
- Bring meals to mourners, to parents of newborns, or sick relatives and friends.

NONHARMING

Right Action is the practice of nonharming. This means not doing anything that hurts yourself, other people, animals, insects, or the environment. Nonharming is a key part of the Eightfold Path. It shows respect for life and acknowledges our interdependence. All of your actions have an impact. Some are helpful to ourselves and others; some are harmful to ourselves and others.

You see this when you take a look at some of your actions and how they make you feel about yourself. If you misuse food day after day, painful feelings are likely to follow. If you treat yourself kindly day after day, you pave the way for self-respect. If you're impatient or rude to a food server—even if you think you're right—you feel guilty later. If you are kind to someone who needs help, you feel good about yourself.

Our actions also have consequences for others and for the world we live in, even if we're not always aware of what they are. One meditation teacher compares the impact of actions to the impact of a small pebble. When it's thrown into a large pond, one tiny pebble creates many ripples, even though it landed on one small spot. It's the same with actions: every action creates ripples that extend in many directions, even though you may not see all of them.

THE IMPACT OF YOUR ACTIONS

All of your decisions regarding food—what you buy and eat, how you cook, and where you shop—have consequences for others. Your family, friends, and community are all affected. For example:

• Recycling bottles, newspapers, and cans reduces the garbage you create.
• Walking to the store reduces air pollution.
• Changing the way you prepare food (e.g., more broiling, less frying) and the types of food you eat (e.g., more grains, less sugar) can improve the health of your family and friends.
• Buying produce at the farmers' market instead of the supermarket can improve the local economy.
• Eating low on the food chain can increase the food supply all over the world.

What's going on in the world also affects you. Most of the time you probably don't think twice about weather conditions around the world, but they appear in your grocery bill from week to week. When there's a drought in Hawaii, you may pass up a pricey fresh pineapple, even though it's a family favorite. A warm summer in central California could mean more green salads because the price of lettuce goes down. An oil spill off Alaska may have impact on the kind of fish you buy. Diseased cows that caused deaths in Britain may trigger a new wave of vegetarianism all over the world.

Practicing Right Action shows respect for this complex chain of actions and consequences: actions in the world affect us, we affect our actions, our actions affect others, and others affect us.

THE UNIVERSE IS ON YOUR PLATE

Vietnamese meditation master Thich Nhat Hanh offers a concrete way to help us appreciate the truth of interdependence with a simple example. He suggests that looking closely at any object, such as a green bean or even this page of paper you're reading, is looking closely at the *entire universe*. How can this be so?

In his poetic style, Thich Nhat Hanh helps us see that there are clouds floating on this page of paper. Without clouds there would be no water; without water, no trees; and without trees, there would be no paper. The existence of this page is dependent on the existence of a cloud. Sunshine is also important because forests can't grow without sunshine and neither can we. So the logger needs sunshine in order to cut a tree and the tree needs sunshine in order to be a tree. Therefore, sunshine is also present on this page. So is the wheat that became bread for the logger to eat. In fact, there's nothing in the universe that is unrelated to this page of paper. The universe contains this page of paper just as this page of paper contains the universe.

Try this exercise yourself. Closely examine a piece of fruit, a bag of garbage, or a few grains of rice. Can you find all of the elements of the universe within these things?

RESPECT FOR LIFE

The Buddha established a monastic order so that men and women could live harmless lives, in harmony with life. Monks and nuns follow precepts called *the Patimokkha Discipline*. These are guidelines for practicing Right Action and are in line with the principles of nonharming. For instance, it is forbidden to intentionally kill anything. Since monastics eat only what is offered to them, they don't kill animals.

The respect monastics show for life goes way beyond not killing. Some monks and nuns don't pick flowers or uproot plants in order not to interfere with the natural flow of life in any way. In Thailand, monastics carry water strainers so that they can filter out living things in the water such as mosquito larvae. That's how careful they are to respect all living things.

Most of us can't imagine living with that level of discipline, mindfulness, or concern for other forms of life. These standards of behavior may appear extreme, but they may not seem so much so when you look at the opposite extreme. Every day millions of animals are slaughtered, forests eliminated, and clean water contaminated to provide food and conveniences that most people take for granted. Think of all the packages, containers, and cans you use and then toss out every day, and multiply that by several million people. The amounts of garbage this creates just in one day is overwhelming.

You don't have to join a monastic community or dramatically change your behavior to practice Right Action. What you do need to do is be mindful of your actions and the impact they have. You may be surprised at how many actions you willingly change the more you reflect on their consequences.

MONASTICS AND
INTERDEPENDENCE

Action and wisdom cannot be separated. It is like using one hand to wash the other. Virtuous actions enable wisdom to shine forth. Wisdom enables action to grow more virtuous. These two qualities are the most precious things in life.
—THE BUDDHA

Monastics live in harmony with the truth of interdependence. They give full recognition to the fact that all lives are interconnected and that we need one another to survive. Monks can't live in complete isolation because it would be too easy to forget this truth. That's why many of the monastic rules ensure that monks depend on others. For instance, monks and nuns can't cook for themselves and they aren't allowed to keep food past noon. These rules compel monastics to be in contact with the community at least once a day so they can receive physical nourishment.

Part of monastic training involves the custom of going on daily alms rounds. Monastics walk through villages with their alms bowls. These bowls represent their dependence on others. Villagers place food in their bowls, which the monastics accept with gratitude. They don't express any preferences about the kinds or amounts of food they are offered. As one monk (and Mick Jagger) said, "You may not always get what you want, but you always get what you need." In some countries people take great joy in giving, even though giving away food was (and is) a big sacrifice. Giving to monastics may mean you and your family eat less.

THE CIRCLE OF GIVING AND RECEIVING

The daily alms round is a symbol of how giving and receiving go both ways: it's a continuous circle of generosity. The monastic and the lay communities offer each other different forms of nourishment. The lay community provides monastics with physical nourishment; the monastics provide the lay community with spiritual nourishment. Both forms of nourishment are essential, and both constitute Right Action.

Daily contact with lay people reminds monastics that their practice is for the benefit of all beings, not just for themselves. As monastics walk through villages and come in contact with the young and old, rich and poor, healthy and sick, they reaffirm their effort to find a way out of the pleasure-seeking, pain-avoiding cycle of suffering. Monastics are indebted to the community for their support. Diligent mindfulness practice is a way of repaying this debt.

For lay people, the alms round is a reminder that happiness and peace of mind are not part of the economy. They're priceless. Monastics embody the values of honesty, loyalty, goodness, and nonharming that are often ignored in the competitive marketplace. The daily alms round also provides lay people with the dignity that comes from being donors.

The Buddha summed up the circle of generosity when he said:

> Monks, householders are very helpful to you. They provide you with the requisites of robes, alms food, lodging, and medicine. And you, monks, are very helpful to householders. You teach them the laws of nature, admirable in the beginning, admirable in the middle, and admirable in the end. In this way the holy life is lived in mutual dependence, for the purpose of crossing over the flood, for making a right end to suffering.

THE CIRCLE OF GRASPING AND SUFFERING

The rules of conduct that monastics live by are designed to support the circle of giving. The opportunities to give and receive are built into the system because they're recognized as important values. This is not the case in most Western cultures. Most people live by rules of conduct that support a circle of grasping. These values stress competition and individualism. Owning a lot of things is a sign of wealth, and bigger usually means better.

Dependence is a sign of weakness. Needing others means you're a drain or that you can't pull your own weight. If others need you, it can trigger fears about not having enough, so you try to accumulate more. The Hungry Ghost takes over by doing what it knows best: wanting more and more only to be satisfied by less and less. And the whole cycle of grasping and suffering goes around and around, gaining more and more strength each time.

There's a folktale that vividly describes how the two kinds of circles generate different kinds of relationships. It's a story about a leader and his three advisors. During one of their discussions, the leader asked, "What is the sweetest melody?"

One advisor answered, "The melody of the flute."

Another disagreed. "It's the melody of the harp that's most beautiful."

The third advisor said, "You're both wrong. The sweetest melody is the violin."

The leader said nothing while the three men argued. Days later, they were still fighting about the right answer to the question. Then it was time to attend a banquet.

Musicians entertained the guests, but there was no food served. Usually, the banquet tables were laden with all kinds of delicacies and sweets. Finally, they let go of the argument. They all wanted to know, "Where's the food?"

At that moment, the leader brought in a large pot of food and beat the side of the pot with a spoon. The sound *clink, clink* resonated throughout the banquet room.

The advisors were smiling and ready to enjoy the food.

Then the leader said, "The clink of dishes in the ears of a hungry person—this is the sweetest melody of all."

The advisors agreed and enjoyed the delicious meal in harmony. This experience taught them a valuable lesson. They weren't being fed while they were arguing; they felt well fed only after they stopped arguing and were in harmony with each other again.

THE GIFT OF FOOD

Every person's blood is red, every person's tears are salty.
—THE BUDDHA

I learn more about interdependence and how the circle of giving and receiving works every time I volunteer in a local soup kitchen. On one level, the difference between my life and the life of the people I feed seems great. On another level, our basic human needs are identical, regardless of color, age, size, shape, gender, nationality, religion, level of education, or income. We all need food, and we all have hunger pangs when we don't eat it.

The people I serve also remind me that hunger and nourishment are part of the same circle of giving and receiving. The hungry people I serve also serve and nourish me. I enjoy the opportunity to reach out beyond my immediate world and help others. My personal problems take on a more balanced perspective. I like the way it feels to hand out plates of hot food to people and see them enjoy their meal. It feels good to give.

The nourishment I receive is different than the nourishment I give, but they're both essential. They are part of the same circle. Everyone's hunger gets satisfied, so in that sense, hungry people are feeding me just as I am feeding them.

When you realize that you're vitally interconnected with everyone, your behavior changes from "What's in it for me?" to "How can I help?"

THREE STORIES OF GENEROSITY

Giving brings happiness at every stage of its expression. We experience joy in forming the intention to be generous; we experience joy in the actual act of giving something; and we experience joy in remembering the fact that we have given.
—MEDITATION TEACHER SHARON SALZBERG

The Gift of Giving

There is a story of two young girls who eat lunch together every day. One eats enormous amounts of food, yet she is never satisfied. The other girl eats moderately and fills up quickly. What's the difference? The first girl's nourishment comes only from what she eats. The other girl's nourishment comes from more than that. Every day she saves some of her lunch and gives it away to someone who's hungry. The giver's sense of fullness doesn't come from how much she's eaten, it's from how much she's given. In return, she feels emotionally full, something no amount of physical food can do.

The Bride's Gift

A story from the Babylonian Talmud shows another kind of gift that comes from generosity. A father learns from an astrologer that his daughter will be bitten by a snake and die on her wedding day. But she survived her wedding day after all.

Her father asked: "How did you escape your prophesied fate?"

She replied, "A poor man came to the door last night asking for some food. Everyone was so busy eating and celebrating, the hungry man was ignored. So I gave him some of my food."

The father realized it was his daughter's generosity that had turned her fate around. Giving a small amount of food to a hungry man meant the woman would receive many more years of life. So inspired by his daughter's good deed and the life-changing consequences of her actions, her father dedicated himself to lecturing on charity's power to deliver from death. The Talmud says that the protective powers of generosity are so strong, they not only protect from an unnatural death but also from death itself.

One Hungry Man

The Buddha was about to begin a talk when he noticed an elderly farmer enter the hall. He could see that the farmer was hungry. Before the Buddha began his talk, he asked that rice and curry be served to the man. Those gathered were restless with impatience. They wondered why they should have to wait to hear the Buddha talk just because of one hungry man.

When the farmer was finished eating, the Buddha said, "Respected friends, if I delivered a talk while our friend was still hungry, he would not be able to concentrate. That would be a pity. There is no greater suffering than hunger. Hunger wastes our bodies and destroys our well-being, peace, and joy. We should never forget those who are hungry. It is a discomfort to miss one meal, but think of the suffering of those who have not had a proper meal in days or even weeks. We must find ways to assure that no one in this world is forced to go hungry."

A RECIPROCAL OPPORTUNITY

Unfortunately, millions of people in this world still go hungry, even though there are enough resources to feed everyone. Probably not far from where you live or work, there are people who don't have enough to eat right now. Hunger affects people of all ages: the elderly, infants, children, teenagers, and adults. Consider these facts:

- Between twenty and thirty million Americans suffer from hunger.
- Half of them are children under twelve.
- Twenty-five million people rely on food pantries, soup kitchens, and other food distribution programs.
- People in one out of ten households receive food stamps.
- The average food stamp benefit is sixty-eight cents per meal.
- Thirty-five thousand to forty thousand children die from hunger every day in Third World countries.

- For the cost of ten Stealth bombers (eight billion dollars a year) hunger in the United States could be eliminated.

Even though the nature of our hunger is different, everyone needs physical and emotional nourishment. The hungry need physical nourishment, like monastics. Those with food obsessions need emotional nourishment, like lay people. Each group has what the other one needs.

Just as the circle of giving feeds monastics and lay people alike, it can also feed those suffering with different forms of hunger. Hungry people need physical nourishment; many food-obsessed people need the emotional nourishment that helping others provides. When there's a circle of giving, everyone gets fed.

Imagine the changes that would take place in the overweight and the hungry alike if an ongoing connection was established between them. If people struggling with the burden of abundance made the commitment to feed the hungry, then both types of hungers could be satisfied. Imagine if this commitment was supported by experts and executives in the food and diet industries. The potential of this aspect of Right Action has yet to be explored.

RIGHT ACTION BEGINS WITHIN

Generosity can't be forced, but it can be practiced. When you feel bad about yourself, it's harder to give. You feel you have nothing worthwhile to offer. You may even resent the pressure to give. But it's important to give, anyway. Your sincere offer to help someone will make a difference to both of you.

If you can't give, examine the reasons why it's so difficult for you. It's good to be honest with yourself about your motivation to help and what you hope to get from it. Make sure you practice being generous toward yourself. When you give to yourself and feel good about it, it's easier to be generous with others.

WAYS TO BECOME MINDFUL OF RIGHT ACTION

Studies show that helping others is emotionally nourishing. People live longer who have pets or who have a living plant to care for. They feel more worthy about themselves than people who live totally independent lives with no responsibilities. Here are some ways you can help and practice Right Action.

1. Experiment with your generosity related to food. Instead of offering spare change to a homeless person, buy the person a piece of fruit, a sandwich, or a beverage.

2. Call the local food bank or Red Cross. Get the names and telephone numbers of places that need assistance.

3. Volunteer in a local soup kitchen or food giveaway program. Feed-the-hungry programs usually operate both throughout the week and on weekends, so finding the right fit with your schedule may be easier than you think.

4. Find out what items are needed most and offer to donate them. Donate fresh food on a regular basis. Dairy

products (milk, eggs, and cheese), fresh fruits, vegetables, and protein sources (such as tuna fish or beans) are usually in demand.

5. Contact local restaurants, bakeries, and supermarkets that have excess food to give away. Offer to deliver it to a feed-the-hungry program or homeless shelter. Catering companies, local businesses, and college cafeterias can also supply food that would otherwise be wasted. Hungry people appreciate the leftovers, there's no wasted food, and there's no additional money involved.

6. Get your friends, relatives, and coworkers involved in feeding the hungry. Instead of going out to eat, volunteer together at a soup kitchen, or pool the money you would have spent eating out and donate it to a program that feeds the hungry.

7. Bring special treats to children in a homeless shelter. Stretch yourself a bit. It feels really good.

CHAPTER 9

RIGHT WAY OF LIVING:

The Power of Integrity

RECIPE #5

◎

And what is Right Way of Living? Refraining from killing,
stealing, false speech, misconduct in relationships, and intoxicants.
This is called Right Way of Living.
—THE BUDDHA

Right Way of Living, the fifth section of the Eightfold Path, means living in a peaceful and dignified way, in harmony with life. This recipe begins within, by giving proper nourishment to both your body and your mind.

Every great spiritual tradition recognizes and teaches basic laws of human conduct. In Buddhism, these laws are called precepts. You may also know them as virtues, ethics, or moral conduct. What they're called doesn't really matter. Their meaning and application, however, matters a lot.

Precepts are guidelines for living without causing harm

to yourself or others. Living by the precepts helps create freedom and happiness, not just in your relationship to food but within your whole life. The precepts include refraining from killing, stealing, misconduct in relationships, harmful speech, and misuse of intoxicants. This recipe shows you how following the precepts helps nourish you so you can enjoy the deep and lasting fullness they offer.

You may be wondering what these precepts have to do with eating. After all, food isn't a religion or spiritual tradition. That's true, but food is crucial to life. It can help sustain or destroy you, everyone you know and love, and every living being on the planet. People kill for food, and millions of others die from not having enough of it.

The precepts alert you to the things that cause a lot of suffering or create a lot of healing for yourself and others. The power of committing to these precepts is enormous, as is the power of not committing to them. Not living by the precepts is often compared to living like a wild beast. You feel consumed by guilt, regret, and self-hatred, and you can do a lot of harm to others. When you're intoxicated by personal desires, there's no alternative voice within you that says, "Wait a minute. Will what I'm about to do cause harm to me or anyone else? Is there any benefit to what I'm about to do?"

Our society is ruled by greed, craving, fear, hatred, and violence. The way to help society is by transforming these passions within ourselves. This, in turn, helps transform the world we live in. For instance: Violence isn't a way to solve problems or your eating challenges. Crash diets are like quick war, where no one really wins. If your intentions are flavored by desire, you help create greed in some form or another.

On the other hand, when you make the effort to live

harmlessly, you can do a lot of good. Your self-respect creates a spirit of generosity around you. By being kind and compassionate toward yourself after an eating binge or toward your overweight body, you are more likely to be kind to yourself as you face other types of challenges. This effect spreads to the way you treat your family, your friends, your colleagues, and the people you meet in stores or on the street. Your willingness to be kind to yourself is the foundation of both inner peace and peace on the planet. Following the precepts not only nourishes you, it nourishes everyone you relate to, and even those you don't relate to.

NOT KILLING: PRECEPT ONE

Killing isn't a matter of taking another life (although it can be). It also means killing parts of ourselves. Food is a typical murder weapon. Maria is the mother of two teenage boys. She has spent a lot of time trying to kill off an important part of her past with food. For the last twenty years, she had been about thirty pounds overweight. She regularly used food to kill memories she didn't want to face. It wasn't until she received a call from a third son—one she had given up for adoption at birth twenty years ago—that she was able to be honest with herself about her eating problems.

Maria always made excuses about why she needed food as a crutch, but her excuses were unrelated to the unexpressed grief she had about giving up an infant. She tried to ward off those painful feelings by stuffing herself with food. After she and her estranged son were reunited, Maria lost thirty pounds and, above all, felt good about herself and her body. She was finally able to be honest about the intense guilt and longing she had for her third son.

Maria has become more sensitive to the importance of practicing the precepts in relationship to eating as a result of this experience. She is committed to being respectful to her feelings, and has made the commitment not to kill off other strong feelings by misusing food. She receives nourishment from the dignity that comes from her commitment to not kill. It gives her the incentive to treat herself gently, especially toward deep feelings of sadness and remorse. Maria can't eliminate her suffering, but following this precept helps change her relationship to it.

The commitment to not killing can be literal. You may want to consider adopting a meatless diet. Not eating meat shows respect to animals, and it also has major health benefits. There's ample evidence to suggest that a nonmeat diet that's filled with a variety of fruits and vegetables may help reduce the risk of cancer, heart disease, and diabetes. In addition, vegetarian diets don't require as many resources as meat-based diets. Instead of growing grain to feed the animals you plan to eat, you just eat the grain. Eating lower on the food chain can affect world hunger. It means there's more food available for everyone. (The distribution of this food is another story.) A healthy vegetarian plan is often less expensive than a meat-based diet, especially when you buy items like oatmeal and rice in bulk, fruits and vegetables in season, and avoid processed, prepared foods, even if they're meatless.

Keep in mind that neither a nonmeat nor a meat-filled diet necessarily will meet your nutritional needs. Everyone needs a balanced diet that includes *a wide variety* of nutritious foods. You can do this as a vegetarian, as a meat eater, or as an occasional meat eater. It's your responsibility to ensure that vital nutrients are included in your diet every day.

NOT STEALING: PRECEPT TWO

The Buddha didn't just encourage eating slowly and listening to the body. He referred to the precept of not stealing when he said: "Let your stomach tell you when to stop, not your eyes or your tongue." You can help yourself do this by breathing in and out as you look at the food on the table, *before you begin to eat*. This gives you the chance to pause and ask, "What is good for my body and what is not?" You can choose what to eat, knowing when you feed yourself, you are feeding and nourishing everyone you know and everyone you don't. In other words, part of the precept of not stealing is a commitment to eating moderately and respectfully.

Stealing isn't just a matter of theft. It can be a metaphor. Acting out strong desires is a form of stealing, like taking more food than you need. It's more nourishing to examine your desire to take more food instead of acting it out. Investigating the desire to get the last dinner roll on the table or to find a way into the front of the food line may reveal important aspects about yourself that need attention. Not stealing also means not stealing attention away from the thoughts, feelings, and situations that need it.

Not stealing is also an opportunity to be grateful and/or generous. It's easier to be generous when you take time to reflect how fortunate you are to have food, shelter, and the luxury to explore why you and others suffer. Acts of generosity bring joy and happiness to others and therefore to yourself. In addition to being more mindful about the quality and quantity of food you eat, make an effort to think about how you want to express generosity and gratitude. All of these actions are wise applications of this precept.

NOT MISUSING FOOD AS AN INTOXICANT: PRECEPT THREE

This precept involves the commitment to cultivate mindful consuming. For many people, this means limiting or abstaining from sugar, caffeine, and alcohol. All of these substances can be used to lift up our spirits or to give us a bolt of energy. There's a big difference however, between enjoying a candy bar during an energetic hike and inhaling several candy bars to numb yourself against anger or other intense feelings. Only you know how much is too much, or whether you should abstain from something altogether.

All of us, however, must realize that these substances can create a lot of suffering when they are misused, especially alcohol. Misusing intoxicants is a betrayal of your body, your family, and everyone who is affected by your actions. It's depleting to feel groggy and listless after a sugar binge or a caffeine high. The amount of money spent on intoxicants of any type can be used for life-affirming acts of generosity. Consider saving the money you ordinarily spend on candy, cookies, coffee, wine, and beer and then donating it to organizations that help others like the local food bank, or the local chapter of Mothers Against Drunk Driving. If you want more immediate and direct gratification, buy nutritious food with the money you save and donate it to a homeless shelter or to a food giveaway program.

Committing to this precept can also include not eating or serving food that contains harmful chemicals and poisons. You may also want to consider restricting or avoiding items that contain a lot of food coloring, nitrates, and preservatives (like certain brands of hot dogs, baked goods, and frozen foods). Make the effort to eat organic fruits and vegetables and whole grains.

MAKE A COMMITMENT TO THE PRECEPTS

There's a lot of nourishment that comes from committing to the precepts. You can tap into a lot of emotional and physical strength within yourself the more you practice them. Take the time to ask yourself:

• What would it mean to eat only things that didn't cause any harm to you or anyone else?
• How can you show love and respect for yourself and others every time you eat?
• What changes do you need to make in order to practice the precepts so that they become the foundation of your life?

Keep in mind that no one can practice the precepts perfectly. Even if you're a vegetarian, the food you eat still contains life, bugs, insects, etc. But practicing the precepts points you in the right direction. It sets up the intention within you to live harmlessly and in harmony with life. Following the precepts can lead to dramatic changes that are needed in ourselves, in our families, communities, and the planet we share.

WAYS TO BECOME MINDFUL OF THE RIGHT WAY OF LIVING

1. Choose one of the five precepts (refraining from killing, stealing, misconduct in relationships, harmful speech, and misuse of intoxicants) and relate it to eating. Commit to practicing it wholeheartedly for at least one month. Continue practicing this precept and then select another precept and practice them both intensively, until you are practicing them all intensively.

• Don't kill your difficult feelings or emotions by eating. Make a commitment to allow painful emotions to come up. Instead of reacting to them, just observe them with kindness and patience. Notice the impulse to kill strong feelings with food and pay close attention to what's driving this need. That's the source of suffering, and that's what needs your attention now.

• Don't steal by taking more food than you need. Make a commitment only to eat when you are hungry. Be moderate in the amount of food you take. Stop every few minutes and check in with how full you feel. Do you need to eat any more? Will you help or hurt yourself by continuing to eat?

• Don't use food as an intoxicant to dull or numb yourself. Make a commitment to restrict your use of eating sugar or caffeine. Both may offer an immediate high, but not without a predictable low. It's more nourishing to learn about the impulse that drives these urges and be patient with yourself in the process.

2. Imagine the impact on yourself and on the world if just *one* precept was followed by every person on the planet. For instance, what would it be like if every food, cosmetic, or weight-loss advertisement told the truth and avoided any and all deceptive practices? What impact would you expect? What impact would you want? How can you help make this happen?

CHAPTER 10

RIGHT EFFORT:
Finding the
Right Balance
RECIPE #6

◎

What is Right Effort? A monk rouses his will, makes an effort, stirs up energy, exerts his mind, and strives to maintain wholesome mind states that have arisen, not to let them fade away, to bring them to greater growth, to the perfection of development. This is called Right Effort.
—THE BUDDHA

The sixth section of the Eightfold Path is Right Effort. This recipe focuses on the energy you put into nourishing yourself. Practicing Right Effort means gathering the energy spent trying to find satisfaction where it can't be found and focusing it on the present moment.

When you practice Right Effort, you see clearly that the endless activity of the mind is exhausting, unsatisfying, and leads to emotional hunger. You recognize that the present moment is what supplies the emotional nourishment you're looking for. It takes effort to remember the truth of impermanence: that a lot of suffering is optional, that the source of happiness and suffering comes from within. There are so many cultural forces (advertisements, movies, television shows, etc.) offering the opposite message: if you buy a certain product, look a certain way, or take a particular vacation, you'll feel satisfied. Desire has a powerful allure when it's well packaged. The ability to walk away from the temptation to satisfy desire after desire takes effort. These messages to buy this and look like that are not commands. You don't have to follow orders blindly like so many of the people did in Milgram's experiments on obedience to authority. You can make the effort to walk away from situations that are harmful or not in your best interest.

FACE SUFFERING AND BECOME FEARLESS

Above all, Right Effort involves a willingness to open to suffering. One Zen master says Right Effort means learning how to become fearless: to have the courage to look at everything without turning away. It takes a lot of emotional strength to face suffering, loneliness, fear, and grief. It also takes effort to face the fact that there are no magical solutions to anything, including managing our physical and emotional appetites. This is why the Buddha said, "A single day's life of useful intense effort is better than a hundred years of idleness and inactivity."

It takes courage to see a feeling clearly for what it is. A lot of what you see are things you don't like: jealousy, resentment, and self-pity. The tendency is to ignore them or to project them onto others. Someone bumps your elbow while you're eating, and you get some salad dressing on your shirt. You think: "Why was he so clumsy? Now I'm going to have a big, ugly stain." You feel furious and you don't enjoy the rest of the meal. You're caught up in anger and you don't even know it. It's difficult to accept your own anger if you believe it's unacceptable, but the more you ignore anger, the more it tends to run your life and keep you feeling hungry for more.

To actually face each moment directly by diving straight into the heart of it is one of the great teachings of Buddhism. Right Effort is not about striving or trying to change anything. It's *letting go of the desire* to change the experience. This special kind of effort has to do with surrender and effort at the same time. It is a continued steadiness in letting go, moment by moment by moment. You let go of how you think things should be or how you want them to be, knowing everything changes on its own. You open to seeing things as they are without adding anything extra.

Things change by bearing with them. If you have a ravenous appetite and want to eat everything in sight, you can make the effort to stay with this experience and not act it out. You allow the feeling to take its course, whatever that may be. The feeling of a ravenous appetite may get stronger and more persistent until you feel you can't stand it anymore, and you bear with those feelings, too. This kind of effort isn't passive acceptance. It's a radical acceptance of learning to bear with something unpleasant until it changes. You don't need to get rid of anything out of aversion. You can let things be and see what happens.

EFFORT AND SURRENDER

Two students of an old rabbi were arguing about the true path to God. One said the path must be built on effort and energy. "You must give yourself totally and fully to follow the way of the law."

The second student disagreed. "It is not effort, it is pure surrender. Letting go is the path to God."

They couldn't agree who was right, so they went to see the rabbi. He listened as the first student praised the path of effort. When he asked the rabbi, "Is this right?" the rabbi said, "Yes, you're right."

The second student got very upset. He argued that it was the path of surrender that was the true path to God. When he finished, he asked the rabbi, "isn't this the true path?" The rabbi responded, "Yes. You're right."

A third student, hearing the discussion, said, "How can they both be right?"

The rabbi responded with a smile. A Zen master would smile, too. Because the nature of this particular kind of effort has to do with letting go, and letting go has to do with acceptance. This radical acceptance of things becomes the path to nourishment. In other words, effort, surrender, and letting go are the same. They belong together and can't happen without one another. In order to cultivate this special kind of effort, it can be very helpful to learn the practice of loving-kindness.

LOVING-KINDNESS

Metta, translated as loving-kindness, is the sincere wish for health and happiness for yourself and others, without exception. It is a benevolent attitude in which you take on a natural empathy. When you are filled with loving-kindness, you cannot harbor ill will toward yourself, toward anyone else, or toward any thing. You see the good and beautiful, not the bad and ugly.

Loving-kindness is the essence of letting go: you make the effort to allow everything to come and go in peace. You allow your Hungry Ghost or your rage to be as they are so they can arise and pass away on their own. You stay centered and balanced within these experiences instead of grasping or rejecting them.

Loving-kindness is a practice, and it's always practiced toward yourself first. The Buddha said that you can search the whole world and never find anyone more worthy of love than yourself. Try a little loving-kindness now. Close your eyes. Take a few deep breaths, and repeat these phrases: "*May I be happy. May I be healthy. May I be peaceful. May I be safe.*"

If any feelings of loving-kindness arise in you, connect the feelings with the phrases. That way they'll become stronger and more familiar to you. If the opposite feelings, such as hatred or anger arise, just observe them. Even these difficult feelings can be flooded with loving-kindness. Be aware of how difficult this may be, and try to be kind to that difficulty, too. Make the effort to be as kind to the difficulties as you would toward the person you cherish the most.

It is a wonderful practice to send loving-kindness toward difficult attitudes and feelings. For instance, if you're feeling frustrated, you can practice *metta* toward this feeling by saying, "May my frustrations be happy. May they be healthy. May they be peaceful. May they be safe." You can direct *metta* toward any feelings or experiences like hating your body or feeling envious of a thin friend.

Loving-kindness may feel strange and unnatural to you, perhaps even fake. All of these feelings can be acknowledged with loving-kindness. Loving-kindness doesn't mean denying these feelings or trying to smooth them over. Like Right Effort, loving-kindness means accepting any kind of feeling so it can arise and pass away naturally. These qualities don't discriminate between good and bad feelings. They allow you to experience the nourishment offered in every moment, regardless of what it is.

WAYS TO BECOME MINDFUL OF RIGHT EFFORT

1. Make the effort to practice loving-kindness every day. Pick a regular time and place (e.g., before breakfast or late afternoon) to practice loving-kindness for a minimum of thirty to sixty minutes. Use this time to send thoughts of loving-kindness to yourself, no matter what mood you are in. Make loving-kindness practice a daily habit, like brushing your teeth or returning telephone calls. In addition to the time you set aside to practice loving-kindness, you can also make it a natural part of your day: Repeat the phrases of loving-kindness as you get dressed, eat, or go to sleep at night.

2. Practice loving-kindness toward your eating challenges. Make the effort to bring an attitude of acceptance toward the tendency to eat mindlessly, judge yourself, or feel impatient, angry, or fearful. What would it take for you to make the effort to let go of these or other difficult experiences?

3. Practice loving-kindness toward others. You may feel inspired to do so for:

- The next waiter or waitress who serves you
- The butcher and produce manager in your supermarket
- The farmers who grow the fruits and vegetables you eat
- Those who package the seeds you plant in your garden
- Every person who had *anything* to do with what you eat today

4. Envision a different world. Imagine how it could be if everyone made the effort to practice loving-kindness every day.

- What impact do you think the practice would have on you, your family, and friends?
- How would it change your behavior toward yourself, the way you eat, the way you relate to others, and how others relate to you?
- Incorporate some of these changes so they become a natural part of your life.

CHAPTER 11

RIGHT MINDFULNESS:

How to Be Here Now

RECIPE #7

◎

And what is Right Mindfulness? Here, monks, a monk abides contemplating body as body, ardent, clearly aware and mindful, he abides contemplating feeling as feelings, he abides contemplating mind as mind, he abides contemplating mind-objects as mind-objects, ardent, clearly aware, and mindful, having put aside hankering and fretting for the world. This is called Right Mindfulness.

—*THE BUDDHA*

Right Mindfulness, the seventh factor of The Eightfold Path, focuses on our natural capacity for observation, investigation, and reflection. This recipe shows how to have *direct insight* into things as they are. It's the key to lasting nourishment.

When done mindfully, an ordinary experience like washing a dirty glass—soaping it up, running hot water over it, drying it sparkling clean—can be perfectly satisfying. If you're really present, you *become* the experience. There's no one washing the glass, there's just washing. This feeling of oneness and the nourishment that it provides can't be found anywhere else but within the present moment. Everything you do, from slicing tomatoes to unpacking the groceries to cleaning up spilled milk, offers this possibility to you when you are mindful.

Ordinary experiences like washing a dirty glass are often overlooked or underrated because the habits of desire are so powerful. Washing a glass doesn't seem as interesting as reading a juicy mystery. If you're trying to wash the glass as quickly as possible so you can get back to reading the book, you're not in the present moment; you're not aware of washing dishes or the fact that you're caught up in think-ing about the future. This is why the Buddha said, *"If you are ruled by thoughts of the past or future, you lose the chance to make real contact with all the wonders of life."* The Buddha isn't suggesting thoughts are a problem, because they are not. He is telling us that being *lost* in thought is the problem. Mindfulness is the solution because it is a chance to make real contact with all the wonders of life.

WASH EACH GLASS MINDFULLY

The principle of mindfulness is very simple. Pay attention to what's happening right now. For instance, when you wash a glass, you know it. If you're lost in thought, you know that, too. You make the effort to continually bring your attention back to whatever is true in that moment.

Part of what is so miraculous about this process is that you see that everything is always changing. You're washing a glass but that experience has many, many parts to it. They're all related to each other and they're always changing.

MINDFULNESS IS TRUSTWORTHY

When you see that change is part of everything, you change, too. You learn that mindfulness is something you can trust. Through mindfulness you learn not to put your trust in fleeting desires that are constantly changing. You learn that no object can either permanently satisfy or permanently frustrate you. You learn that clinging creates hunger and that letting go creates nourishment. You know these things directly because you experienced them.

HOW TO BE MINDFUL OF
STANDING IN LINE

Consider the common experience of waiting in line at the grocery store. How can you become more mindful of it? This experience isn't particularly joyful. If there are many people ahead of you, it's easy to get irritated. It's your bad luck to stand behind someone in the quick checkout line who has fifteen items. You wish people would read the sign that says TWELVE ITEMS OR LESS. Your mind feels scrambled as it flips from one disturbed thought to another.

You can turn this situation around by being mindful of

what's going on. There's a whole world of things for you to observe just within your body. As you stand in line, scan your body. Notice the primary sensations that are present. Be aware that you are standing and feel your feet on the ground. What sensations are present? How long can you stay with each of them? You can also notice your breath within the body. Feel yourself breathing in and out through your mouth or nose. Is the breath deep or shallow? Long or short? It can be very relaxing to just feel the upper and lower lips resting on each other as you breathe.

Paying attention to your breath and body may sound dull at first, but it's only because you're not used to being in the present. The more you practice being in the present, the more interested you will become in it. There's a whole world for you to explore that's available right now.

Standing in line at the grocery store can also be an opportunity to enjoy the scent of citrus from the oranges in your shopping cart or to send *metta* (loving-kindness) to yourself. You can turn this mundane and often irritating experience into an opportunity to be mindful. It's a lot easier to be mindful of irritation than it is to mindlessly generate more reasons to feel irritated.

DON'T WASTE VALUABLE MOMENTS JUDGING YOURSELF

There's another important way that mindfulness practice creates change within you. It prevents you from wasting valuable moments that otherwise are spent beating yourself up or putting yourself down. When you look mindfully at your thoughts, it's amazing to realize how many of them are self-critical. We're constantly judging and berating ourselves, rather than mindfully noting this tendency. For instance, you feel bad that you ran out of juice the last time your friends were over, and you can't stop thinking about how stupid you were not to buy enough. That thought spins out to other angry thoughts about all the other things you don't like about yourself, and the whole day gets ruined. When you mindfully acknowledge "Judging," and return to what's going on, you can limit this self-criticism and therefore limit the suffering it creates.

STEPHANIE'S STRUGGLE

Stephanie and her sister have had a close relationship. Stephanie just found out that her sister has a rare blood disease. When she got the news of her sister's illness, the first thought that came to her mind was, "Maybe I'll lose some weight. The last time I got upset, I lost twenty pounds."

Stephanie was shocked by these thoughts and then got angry at herself. "What a selfish person I am. How can I think about losing weight when my sister is so sick?" She experienced her thoughts as "mine," instead of being mindful of them.

Once she became mindful of anger toward herself, Stephanie could return her focus of attention back to her sister. She didn't waste precious time or energy making herself feel worse.

GATHAS

Gathas are short verses that you can recite during the day to help you attend to the present moment. When you focus your mind on a *gatha*, you return to yourself and become more aware of what you're doing. When the *gatha* ends, you can continue what you're doing with heightened awareness. For instance, as you're looking at food, you can recite, "*This plate of food, so fragrant and appetizing, also contains suffering.*" When you're hearing sounds, you can recite, "*Listen, listen, this wonderful sound brings me back to my true self.*"

Like loving-kindness, *gathas* can be said any time or any place because you say them silently. It's really a beautiful practice to acknowledge what you're doing. It brings a sense of the sacred to your life, rather than experiencing your life as one routine task (or errand) after another. Even throwing out the garbage can be an opportunity to reflect on the nature of life and bring you back to the sacredness of the moment. Garbage can smell terrible, especially when it's rotting. I remember living in New York City during one of the garbage strikes. The smell in the streets was absolutely disgusting, and no one could get away from it. Then someone suggested thinking about garbage as compost for beautiful flowers, fruits, and vegetables. Realizing that garbage helps create these things helped me turn my attention away from the stink of rotting garbage to thoughts about the interconnectedness of everything and everyone.

Thich Nhat Hanh has written a book called *Present Moment Wonderful Moment*, which is a collection of mindfulness verses for daily living. There are *gathas* about many things you do every day that you tend not to notice: looking at your hand, taking a bath, driving a car, scrubbing vegetables, and even cleaning the bathroom. I highly recommend incorporating some of these *gathas* into your life as a way of reinforcing mindfulness practice. You can also create your own verses that match the particular circumstances of your daily life, so you feel a more intimate connection to them.

ESTABLISH A DAILY MINDFULNESS PRACTICE

It's impossible for me to emphasize enough the importance of a daily mindfulness practice, one in which you take time to sit in silence and train your mind to attend without clinging to the present moment. Set aside a certain time and place to practice each day. Allow nothing to stand in your way of this time alone, even if it means getting up earlier or staying up later, or drastically rearranging your daily schedule.

Here are the basic instructions:

As you sit, feel the sensations in your body. Notice what sounds, feelings, thoughts, etc., are present. Allow them all to come and go, to rise and fall like ocean waves. Just rest in the midst of these waves. In the center of the waves, feel your breathing. Let your attention feel the in breath and then the out breath. Relax and rest your attention on each breath in any rhythm, long or short, shallow or deep. Let everything else go. When you notice that your mind has wandered, acknowledge it softly and give it a name, such as remembering, restless, wanting. Then return to the breath. Notice that certain thoughts or feelings are pleasurable or painful, and just let them be. After you have sat for between thirty and sixty minutes, open your

eyes and look around before getting up. As you move, try to allow the
same spirit of awareness to go with you into the activities of your day.
Be kind to yourself and let things come and go.

Ultimately, this practice is the foundation of self-
nourishment. Everything that you do to nourish yourself
grows from this. A daily sitting practice is necessary if you
really want to learn the art and skills of self-nourishment,
but sitting daily isn't easy for a number of reasons. Above
all, it can be a challenge to just sit and watch your mind.
You get bored, you don't like what you see, you feel uncomfortable with your posture. All of these things do and
will come up. But you can learn to make peace with them.
Everything is part of the path. If you can learn to resist the
temptation to get up and go for a walk instead, you are
planting the seeds to resist the temptation to eat extra food
or to eat when you're not hungry. If you can learn to accept
feelings of loneliness while you meditate, you're less likely
to act out these feelings by overeating in other situations.
In order words, a daily sitting practice helps build inner
strength and it's this inner strength that helps nourish you
throughout your life.

Give yourself the gift of a committed practice. Make a
commitment to it as if your life depended on it, because it
does. You are being offered a very precious opportunity,
but only you can take it. Make this investment in yourself
just as the Buddha did 2,500 years ago. You can't reap the
benefits of the Four Noble Truths and experience the self-
nourishment that's within unless you make the commitment
to train your mind. Slow down long enough to see your
habitual patterns of behavior. By observing these patterns
and the tendency to grasp or reject your experience, you
are deconditioning the mind from the source of suffering.

This is how you create the experience of nourishment. It's the absence of grasping that creates the loving, nourished heart.

WAYS TO BECOME MINDFUL OF RIGHT MINDFULNESS

1. Bring mindful awareness to the following activities. Pay attention to the thoughts in your mind and to the feelings and sensations in your body as you pour a glass of water, peel a carrot, open and close the refrigerator, and eat one bite of food at a time.

• When your mind has wandered, bring your attention back to the activity.
• How long can you stay with each experience?
• What changes do you notice after mindfully doing these things for a week? A month? Six months? A year?

2. Establish a regular mindfulness practice.

• Pick a regular time (a minimum of thirty to sixty minutes a day) and a quiet place.
• Commit to watching one predominant experience (your breath, your feelings, your thoughts) and return to it each time your mind wanders.
• Encourage your friends and family to establish their own practices, or invite people to practice with you.
• Find out about meditation classes or a mindfulness-based stress-reduction workshop in your area, or consider going on a meditation retreat. Please consult the resource list in the back of the book for more information.

CHAPTER 12

RIGHT CONCENTRATION:
Turning Obstacles Into Opportunities

RECIPE #8

◎

What is Right Concentration? Here, a monk is detached from sense-desires, with inner tranquillity, remaining imperturbable, mindful and clearly aware, beyond pleasure and pain, and purified by equanimity and mindfulness, remains in a concentrated state filled with delight and joy. This is Right Concentration. And that, monks, is called the way of practice leading to the cessation of suffering.
—THE BUDDHA

The eighth section of the Eightfold Path is Right Concentration. This recipe is the culmination of what you've learned along the way. Right Concentration is the ability to sustain mindful attention, moment to moment, without getting derailed by desire. This skill creates a continuity of mindfulness that allows you to fully experience the moment just as it is. Right Concentration is deeply satisfying because it steadies the mind and heart so you can receive the nourishment the moment has to offer.

You have to look deeply at things *over time* in order to see them clearly. It's not just a simple matter of taking a quick look at your Hungry Ghost or memorizing the phrases of loving-kindness. When you sustain your attention, you penetrate the moment instead of staying outside it. This focused awareness helps you see that nothing is concrete and that everything changes. This is a tremendously liberating insight. It helps you see the futility of grasping or rejecting anything. It's just a moment arising and passing away.

The *object* of attention isn't important. It can be a piece of fruit worthy of a Bonnard painting or a rotten, smelly banana peel headed for the compost heap. With sustained mindfulness, you receive nourishment from the intimacy that comes from awareness in any moment, regardless of its content.

When there is sustained awareness of the present moment, gratitude, generosity, and compassion arise as does the willingness to align yourself with the highest and most compassionate standards of conduct. There's no higher form of nourishment than this. You taste the sweet nectar of life purely.

Right Concentration is a practice like everything else on this path. It takes great determination and perseverance to bring your attention back to the present moment again and again: Here's chewing, here's tasting, here's swallowing, here's forgetting, here's the breath, here's hating. This takes effort because the habit of the mind is to be in constant motion, grasping at this or rejecting that. Even within a fairly concentrated state of awareness, it's quite amazing to observe the subtle (and not so subtle) movements of desire. In one moment, you feel totally at one with the apple you are chewing, and in the next moment you're wondering if you're going to like the food served during your next vacation.

Through practicing Right Concentration, you learn to transform the forces of desire into sources of nourishment. Thich Nhat Hanh, the Vietnamese monk and meditation master says, "When you look deeply and mindfully, you see the garbage and the rose. Good organic gardeners do not discriminate against compost, because they know how to transform it into roses." That's the challenge of Right Concentration. How can you turn obstacles into opportunities without grasping or rejecting anything?

Hindrances are the obstacles that make it difficult for you to continue the path of mindfulness. They can either cause tremendous suffering or create an opportunity to open your heart. Self-hatred can be a gateway to compassion or a living hell. Cutting vegetables can be a bloody bore or a fascinating adventure. How they are perceived depends on your relationship to them.

Desire is the most common hindrance. It takes you away from mindfulness by tantalizing you with unrealized possibilities: the desire to try a new restaurant or order a pizza. You feel driven to look elsewhere for nourishment. That desire is not a problem; it's the lack of awareness that cuts you off from the nourishment offered within the moment.

Aversion is another common hindrance. You get derailed by things you don't like. For instance, you are focused on mixing a salad and suddenly you feel irritated. You don't like wasting your time in the kitchen. You have more important things to do. This feeling of aversion has diverted your attention from the present moment.

Restlessness is the hindrance that creates that uneasy, tense feeling that makes you feel like nibbling at food. It's a distraction from what's really going on in the moment, which is the unsettled and unrecognized feeling of restlessness within you.

Laziness is the hindrance that says, "Don't bother to make an effort." It's a sluggish feeling that might be compared to dragging around a heavy sack of potatoes on your back.

Doubt is the hindrance that says, "Mindfulness doesn't work. It's not all that it's cracked up to be. I think I'm going to try another 1,200-calorie-a-day diet."

MILAREPA'S METHOD

Milarepa was a man who lived in a cave by himself and meditated wholeheartedly for years. If he couldn't find anything to eat, he'd eat nettles. But he never stopped practicing mindfulness. One evening, he returned to his cave and found it filled with demons (hindrances). They were cooking his food (the demons of desire), sleeping in his bed (the demons of laziness), and rearranging his belongings (the demon of aversions). They had taken over. Determined to continue his mindfulness practice, Milarepa considered how he was going to get these demons out of the cave. He was aware that the demons were a projection of his own mind, a projection of all of the unwanted parts of himself, yet he didn't know how to get rid of them.

He tried a number of things. He taught the demons how

to meditate; he told them about the power of compassion, the oneness of life, and the importance of generosity. But they were all still there. Then he lost his patience, and he got angry. Then they got angry. Others just laughed and went right back to what they were doing.

Finally he surrendered, sat down on the floor of the cave, and said, "I give up. Let's just live here together." In that moment of surrender, they all left except the one demon he was hoping would be the first to leave. This demon really bugged him; he was particularly nasty and sarcastic. At that point, Milarepa didn't know what to do. Out of sheer desperation, he put his head in the mouth of the demon and said, "Eat me if you want to." It was an act of total surrender, a willingness to completely let go of wanting to change the situation. In that moment of acceptance and surrender, the demon vanished.

Milarepa's method and message are important ones. When your resistance to each moment is gone, so are the demons. You can't trick them into leaving or try to sweet-talk them out of your life. You have to learn to relax and surrender to them. That's the practice of Right Concentration.

TERRY'S METHOD

Terry spent years riddled with anxiety. In everyday language, she was a nervous wreck. There was no peace in her relationship to anxiety; she hated the feelings that drove her to overeat, make a lot of telephone calls, and begin reading books that she never finished. When Terry first began to practice mindfulness, she meditated for about five minutes and then would jump up to make a cup of tea or put on the radio. She was ready to give up on meditation and mindfulness practice when her meditation teacher suggested, "Just notice the hindrance of restlessness every time it comes up."

So that's what Terry did for many months. She noted restlessness in every aspect of her life, from the moment she woke to the moment she went to sleep and throughout her daily mindfulness practice. At first, Terry noticed the way she said "Restlessness" to herself. The tone of her inner voice was filled with seething hatred. After a few months, she noticed a change in that inner voice. It had changed from an angry, hissing tone to a very blasé one: "Oh there's restlessness," as if she was noticing the toothpaste on the side of the sink. Restlessness had lost its charge. She still felt certain feelings in her body and thoughts in her mind that she recognized as restlessness, but they didn't drive her away from whatever she was doing. Terry learned to coexist with restlessness, realizing that it comes and goes on its own when she doesn't struggle against it. Like Milarepa, Terry invited her demon to live with her. As a result of this act of kindness, her entire relationship to restlessness changed.

There are many ways to deal with hindrances. All of these methods are forms of letting go, surrender, loving-kindness, and nourishment at the same time. In the moment you give up the struggle, it becomes a source of nourishment once again. Here are some suggestions for you to apply as you practice turning obstacles into opportunities.

WAYS TO BECOME MINDFUL OF
RIGHT CONCENTRATION

1. Be forgiving toward your hindrances. Forgiveness enables you to soften to obstacles instead of hardening against them. Say to yourself, "It's not easy, but I forgive these hindrances. They're part of being alive." Even if you don't *feel* forgiving, you can still make an effort. You can imagine the hindrance in the form of a neglected, screaming infant in need of being held and nurtured. How can you hold your hindrances with this level of care? Use whatever kind of image opens you and enables you to bring forgiveness to your struggle.

2. Put the hindrance in perspective. Ask yourself:

• At the end of my life, how much will it really mean to me to fulfill this desire (e.g., eating this cookie; attending another cooking class)?

• Will I even *remember* this situation in a few months or years from now?

• Remind yourself that no matter how many times you get what you want, lasting nourishment has nothing to do with fulfilling desire after desire. It has to do with making peace with the forces that are driving these desires.

3. Magnify the hindrances. Try the Milarepa method and let it overcome you. Want, love, or hate as powerfully as you can. Don't act them out, just feel them in your body

and mind. *When you deliberately* amplify the experience, you penetrate it. As the painter Cezanne said, "Exaggerate for a deeper effect." Put your head in the mouth of:

- *Wanting* a piece of cake more than anything else in the world
- *Hating* plain tofu
- *Loving* raisin bread and cream cheese (or fill in your favorite food)
- *Dreading* putting on a bathing suit
- *Believing* mindfulness is a bore
- *Needing* reassurance that you're lovable

Above all, make the commitment to look deeply and mindfully at what gets in the way of sustained awareness. Any obstacle is an opportunity for nourishment. Every obstacle is a compost heap ready to become a rose, just as a rose is certain to become part of a compost heap at some time or another. Practice putting your head in the mouth of whatever demon appears, and see what happens.

CONCLUSION:
Free at Last?

These words are simple. Mastering them is hard.
—TAO TE CHING

No matter where you are on this path, nourishment is always possible when you use the present moment as your guide.

The Four Noble Truths help us see that the present moment is a gift. It comes in many shapes, forms, and sizes: as a body, a meal, a feeling, a fear, or a menu. The First Noble Truth teaches us to see the gift clearly, to be aware of its impermanent nature. The Second Noble Truth teaches us to understand our relationship to this gift. Grasping to make it stay longer or rejecting it, hoping it will go away faster, is what creates suffering. The Third Noble Truth teaches that inner peace comes from learning to let go of the fight. The Fourth Noble Truth describes the Eightfold Path. It teaches you the priceless gift of nourishing yourself in ways that provide lasting food for your heart.

You don't become enlightened; it's something you already are. There are no weight-loss experts who can give you freedom from suffering. You are the one and only authority. Only you can practice the skills that are part of this path. Only you can look within, observe, investigate, and let go.

You can read the Four Noble Truths and the different aspects of the Eightfold Path again and again, but unless you apply them, the words don't really matter. As it says in the Chinese text, *Tao Te Ching*, "These words are simple. Mastering them is hard." It's not about agreeing with these truths or thinking, "They sound pretty good to me." You have to *realize* them in every moment, while you're slicing a tomato or sealing a Ziploc plastic bag.

Your awareness of the present is the nourishment you've been looking for. The opportunity to be aware is fleeting. Meals come and go. The smell of fresh chocolate chip cookies arises and passes away. Ice cream melts. Crunchy vegetables eventually become limp. The chocolate on your child's cheek gets wiped off. Notice these gifts as they appear, knowing that they will change.

WHEN I OVEREAT

Sometimes I get frustrated when I see myself overeating or notice that I've gained weight. Then I stop to remind myself that the Buddha was a human being just as I am. He practiced mindfulness as I must practice it. There are no shortcuts. It's not possible to skip any of the steps. You can't skip learning about suffering through attachment to desire, nor can you skip learning how to be generous to yourself and others.

Every aspect of the path needs to be examined thoroughly. It's useful to think of the first three Noble Truths as the principles of good cooking and nourishing eating. While it may be impossible to fully manifest these principles in every moment, you can keep practicing them for the rest of your life. Refining your speech, practicing generosity and loving-kindness, and being present for the sensations in your body aren't things you can ever overdo.

In every moment, a new set of ingredients is being offered to you. Those ingredients have never been here before, and they'll never be here again. What you create is up to you. It doesn't necessarily matter if the recipe turns into a success or a flop, because whatever gets created in one moment changes in the next one.

I recently learned that when the Buddha went on his first alms rounds, he threw up. Call me weird, but I love that story. I love it because the Buddha had such a natural response to an unfamiliar situation. The food that was offered made him sick to his stomach. It was so different from the food he had received as a prince. It's an experience I can easily identify with. But that experience didn't prevent the Buddha from pursuing the path to freedom. He didn't give up his quest for inner peace because he didn't like the food. He persisted and practiced receiving each moment as it unfolded, regardless of its contents. That's what you and I must do, too. We need to become intimate with the hindrances, make friends with Mara, and spend time with the Hungry Ghost.

As I mentioned in the introduction, I was forced to surrender to many aspects of my life. Within a brief period of time, I had to let go a lot. This letting go included several people who were very precious to me and my work as a psychologist and with Dieters Feed the Hungry. About all I could do was sleep. Not surprisingly, I also gained a lot of weight. The thyroid medication I was taking slowed down my metabolism, and I had hardly any energy for physical activity.

What got me through this emotionally sad and physically difficult time was a commitment to the Four Noble Truths and a daily mindfulness practice. I brought my attention back to them again and again. I saw everything through the lens of these truths, including my tired, flabby body and sad heart. I felt resistance and resentment. I saw frustration and a lot of fear. When I was finally able to accept these feelings, I realized that feeling them was a lot easier than trying to pretend they didn't exist or wishing they would all go away. But all of this took practice.

Things have changed. A lot of my energy has returned, and I've lost weight. I'm back at work. But I know that things will change again. The awareness that things change has given me a sense of security and confidence I never had before.

You don't need to get sick or experience loss to gain this security and confidence for yourself. Just practice every day and commit to using the Four Noble Truths as your anchor. They are never out of date. They are always relevant: there's suffering, a cause, a way out, and a path that shows the way out. That formula will never change.

People often ask me, "What's the bottom line for losing

weight and keeping it off?" I used to suggest things like regular exercise or eating a variety of foods in moderation. Now I only suggest practicing the recipes for nourishing the heart. That's how you learn to be kind to yourself and to every moment. You can spend the rest of your life practicing how to receive the moment with kindness and your time will be well spent.

Joseph Goldstein, a highly respected meditation teacher, emphasizes the importance of setting a time to practice mindfulness every day. He says that if it were possible, he'd implant a subliminal message in people that says, "Practice every day. Practice every day. Practice every day." I want to reinforce that message to you. Establishing a daily practice and commiting yourself to it is essential. Just as brushing your teeth every day is something you do naturally and automatically, you need to establish the same relationship to training your mind. Don't fool yourself into believing that a long walk or listening to music serves the same purpose. They do not. You can certainly bring mindfulness to these situations. This is not the same as training the mind to look deeply at the nature of all things. This is not the same as training the mind to stay present without grasping. This is not the same as training the mind to be kind.

A daily practice is the only way you can really learn how to be kind. Offer yourself the challenge to learn how to be kind to anything: hatred, jealousy, or the feeling of being sick to your stomach. One of the greatest lessons of my life was learning to be kind to intense feelings of hatred and rage I had toward someone. This was my practice for a long time. After many years, that person and I attended the same event and when we saw each other, we spontaneously embraced. I feel tremendous gratitude toward this person for offering me the opportunity to look deeply at my own feelings of hatred and to practice being kind toward it. The feeling of hatred in this situation is long gone. It will probably return in another situation. But that's life. As long as I can practice kindness toward hatred, hatred can't hurt me or anyone else.

When you practice kindness for yourself, you're practicing it for everyone, and everyone who practices it also practices kindness for you. The more you practice kindness, the more you, your family and friends, and the planet we share are nourished by it.

I'll end this book with some of the words with which I began: What you eat or don't eat is not what counts. The key to healthy eating is learning how to change your state of mind. This book is an invitation to look within, and that invitation is always open to you. Food for the heart provides the only kind of nourishment that lasts. So make the commitment to practice every day: Be mindful, be kind, be generous, be grateful, and learn to let things be.

Follow the 2,500-year-old recipe called the Four Noble Truths. Practice every day. Then feast on the nourishment that's available in every moment.

May you and all beings always have enough to eat.
May the circle of nourishment remain unbroken.

USEFUL BOOKS AND
RESOURCES

Aitken, Robert, *The Mind of Clover: Essays in Zen Buddhist Ethics.* Northpoint Press, 1984.

Berg, Frances, *Afraid to Eat: Children and Teens in Weight Crisis.* HWJ, 1997.

Boorstein, Sylvia, *It's Easier Than You Think.* HarperSanFrancisco, 1996.

Brown, Edward Espe, *Tomato Blessing and Radish Teachings: Recipes and Reflections.* Riverhead Books, 1997.

Feldman, Christina, and Jack Kornfield, *Stories of the Heart, Stories of the Spirit.* HarperSanFrancisco, 1991.

Glassman, Bernard, and Rick Fields, *Instructions to the Cook.* Bell Tower Books, 1996.

Hanh, Thich Nhat, *Being Peace.* Parallax Press, 1987.

Hanh, Thich Nhat, *The Heart of Understanding.* Parallax Press, 1988.

Hanh, Thich Nhat, *Present Moment Wonderful Moment*, Parallax Press, 1990.

Hanh, Thich Nhat, *Touching Peace*. Parallax Press, 1992.

Hyde, Lewis, *The Gift: Imagination and the Erotic Life of Property*. Vintage Books, 1983.

Kabat-Zinn, Jon, *Full Catastrophe Living*. Delta, 1990.

Kabat-Zinn, Jon, *Wherever You Go, There You Are*. Hyperion, 1994.

Kornfield, Jack, *A Path with Heart*. Bantam, 1993.

Lao Tzu, *Tao Te Ching*. Penguin, 1986.

Marc, David, *Nourishing Wisdom*. Bell Tower Books, 1992.

Milgram, Stanley, *Obedience to Authority*. Harper and Row, 1974.

Salzberg, Sharon, *Loving-kindness: The Revolutionary Art of Happiness*. Shambala, 1995.

Schwartz, Hillel, *Never Satisfied: A Cultural History of Diets, Fantasies and Fat*. The Free Press, 1986.

Vegetarian Times, *Everything You Need to Know to Be a Healthy Vegetarian*. Macmillan, 1996.

Wallace, B. Alan, *Tibetan Buddhism from the Ground Up*. Wisdom, 1993.

SELECTED RESOURCES

For information on learning meditation at home, write to: Correspondence Course by Sharon Salzberg and Joseph Goldstein (eighty-eight-page workbook and twelve audiocassettes, $198.00)

Sounds True
P.O. Box 8019
Boulder, CO 80306
(800)333-9185

For information on mindfulness-based stress-reduction programs, write to:

Indriya's Net:
The Bulletin of Mindfulness-Based Stress-Reduction Network
Center for Mindfulness
University of Massachusetts Medical Center
Worcester, MA 01655-0267

Subscriptions are $24 annually.

For free books on Buddhism and meditation, write to:

Abhayagiri Monastery
16201 Tomki Road
Redwood Valley, CA 95470

Insight Meditation Society
Pleasant Street
Barre, MA

For more information about meditation, write to:

Spirit Rock
P.O. Box 909
Woodacre, CA 94973

For a catalog of tapes of talks on Buddhism or guided loving-kindness meditations, write to:

Dharma Seed Tape Library
P.O. Box 66
Wendell Depot, MA 01380

For more information and articles on meditation and schedule of retreats and events, write to:

Inquiring Mind
P.O. Box 9999
Berkeley, CA 94709

A donation-supported semiannual journal

INDEX

Abstinence, to control desire, 40–41
Acting out, 145
Action
  and wisdom, 130
  See also Right Action
Addiction, food as intoxicant, 146,
  148–149
Advertising, false claims, 122–123
Alms, for monastics, 131
Attachment to desire
  and abstinence, 40–41
  danger aspect, 50–52
  and fear, 44
  getting rid of, 41–42
  Hungry Ghost, 38–40, 42, 44, 52
  identifying desires, 41
  and identity, 45–49
  meaning of, 36–37
  mindfulness of, 52–53
  versus preferences, 44–45
  relationship to attachment,
    exploring, 64
  and suffering, 45, 47
  See also Letting go

Aversion, versus mindfulness, 171–
  172
Avoidance desires, meaning of, 41

Beauty, appreciation of, 85
Becoming desires, meaning of, 41
Bodhi tree, 7
Buddha, life of, 6–8

Change, mindfulness of, 31
Choice, overabundance of, 94–
  95
Comfort food, 102–103
Common Grace, 109
Concentration. *See* Right
  Concentration
Consumers, information sources
  for, 123
Craving. *See* Attachment to desire
Critical speech, 118–120

Dedication of merit, 103–104
  examples of, 103–104
Dependence, 133